Computed Tomography of the Eye and Orbit

Computed Tomography of the Eye and Orbit

Steven B. Hammerschlag, M.B.B.Ch., F.R.C.P.(C.)

Assistant Clinical Professor of Radiology
University of California, San Francisco
Radiologist, Providence Hospital, Oakland, California
Formerly, Assistant Professor of Radiology, Harvard Medical School;
Neuroradiologist, Brigham & Women's and Beth Israel Hospitals, Boston, Massachusetts

John R. Hesselink, M.D.

Assistant Professor of Radiology
Harvard Medical School
Neuroradiologist, Massachusetts General Hospital, Boston, Massachusetts

Alfred L. Weber, M.D.

Associate Professor of Radiology
Harvard Medical School
Chief of Radiology
Massachusetts Eye & Ear Infirmary, Boston, Massachusetts

APPLETON-CENTURY-CROFTS/Norwalk, Connecticut

83 84 85 86 87 / 10 9 8 7 6 5 4 3 2 1

Prentice-Hall International, Inc., London
Prentice-Hall of Australia, Pty. Ltd., Sydney
Prentice-Hall of India Private Limited, New Delhi
Prentice-Hall of Japan, Inc., Tokyo
Prentice-Hall of Southeast Asia (Pte.) Ltd., Singapore
Whitehall Books Ltd., Wellington, New Zealand
Editora Prentice-Hall do Brasil Ltda., Rio de Janeiro

Library of Congress Cataloging in Publication Data

Hammerschlag, Steven B.
    Computed tomography of the eye and orbit.

    Bibliography: p.
    Includes index.
    1. Eye—Radiography.   2. Eye-sockets—Radiography.
3. Tomography.   I. Hesselink, John R.   II. Weber,
Alfred L.   III. Title. [DNLM: 1. Tomography, X-ray
computed.   2. Orbit—Radiography.   3. Eye—Radiography.
WW 143 H224c]
RE79.R3H26 1983   617.7′1572   82-16257
ISBN 0-8385-1194-5

Design: Jean M. Sabato

PRINTED IN THE UNITED STATES OF AMERICA

To Debra, Ilse, and Patricia
Kay and André
Gloria and Rachael

Contents

Foreword

It was not long after the discovery of x-rays by Roentgen in 1895 that they were used to obtain images of the skull. I am sure that Arthur Schüller of Vienna was one of the first to become involved in the radiography of the orbit in view of his interest in radiography of the skull and facial structures. He published a book on radiology of the skull in 1906, which was translated into English and published in 1912. Some time in the late 1920s or early 1930s, radiography of the orbits was employed to study traumatic and neoplastic lesions. A method was also described to accurately localize radiopaque foreign bodies in their relationship to the globe. There was no other method to visualize the soft tissues of the orbit until the introduction of orbital pneumography. The combination of tomography with orbital pneumography yielded fairly good detail of the anatomy of the orbit. It was, however, technically difficult to control the exact placement of the air and this modality did not become generally or frequently utilized. Surgeons preferred orbital exploration for removal of tumors, determining the relationship of the lesion to the normal structures at the operating table.

The visualization of the eye and other orbital structures was achieved in the late 1950s with the introduction of orbital ultrasound. For the first time it was possible to see the soft tissues within the eye as well as the area around the eye up to the bony walls. The high-resolution ultrasound beam yielded excellent detail in many conditions and still has some advantages over computed tomography. However, it was not until the development and technical improvements of the latter technique that exploration of the orbit by means of cross-sectional imaging techniques reached its present state of development.

With this work the authors hope to present a state-of-the-art approach to the diagnosis of orbital lesions by cross-sectional imaging techniques. This book is intended for students and specialists in both imaging diagnosis and ophthalmology. This I believe the authors have achieved.

Juan M. Taveras, M.D.

Preface

The successful application of computed tomography is exemplified by the major role it has assumed in the diagnosis of orbital pathology. Except for vascular diseases, it has virtually replaced invasive diagnostic modalities such as angiography and venography. The clarity of presentation of orbital structures by computed tomography (CT) has prompted investigations into detailed multiplanar anatomy of the orbit. Tumor margins and inflammatory processes are so clearly defined that one can place the lesions in specific compartments and accurately determine the extent of the disease processes. Orbital involvement by extra-orbital diseases are also well delineated. Specific CT criteria have been established to assist in differential diagnosis.

With the increasing utilization of CT in orbital diagnosis, radiologists have been confronted with a new spectrum of disorders, many of which did not enter the radiology department prior to the advent of CT. The situation is compounded by the fact that orbital disease accounts for a small part of the average CT scanner load and therefore provides little opportunity for one to gain expertise in this area.

It was our aim, therefore, to consolidate our accumulated experience in a concise book which would serve as a reference for the occasional diagnostic dilemma and also provide a general review of all the major disease entities affecting the orbit. We have introduced each chapter with a brief text describing pathology, salient clinical features and the CT findings of each disease. We have also included references for more in-depth reading. The case history format provides a clinical bias to the illustrated material, including follow-up and surgical findings in many cases. It is our hope that this aspect will purvey a broader perspective to the disorders discussed, and will be particularly useful to ophthalmologists.

Acknowledgments

We could not have undertaken this project without the support of our many colleagues and assistants. We are especially indebted to Dr. Roy Strand of the Children's Hospital Medical Center in Boston, who generously provided us with numerous pediatric cases. A special acknowledgment is also made to Karen Easter, research assistant at the Massachusetts Eye and Ear Infirmary for her invaluable contribution.

We are grateful to all of our colleagues, both radiologists and ophthalmologists, who sent us cases either as patients for scanning or as completed images. In this regard we wish to thank the following: Drs. Reed Altemus, Richard Baker, Donald Bienfang, Richard Dallow, Arthur Grove, Susan Hughes, Thornton Kell, Gregory Krohel, Simmons Lessell, Glyn Lloyd, Dan O'Leary, Gerald O'Reilly, Keith Richards, David Walton, and Charles Wright. In addition, we obtained valuable advice from Dr. Richard Dallow, especially in regard to the chapter on Inflammatory Disease.

We wish to thank CT technologists Carolyn Pickett, Brian Chiango, Warren Benson, Margaret Raymond, and Robert Gately for their effort, and Jackie Solberg, Anna Tyas, Claudia Violetta, Linda Fieldhouse, Susan Olsen, Diane Langone, and Denise Festa for their secretarial assistance. A special acknowledgment is made to Don Sucher, who labored meticulously with the photography. Recognition is also given to Harriet Greenfield, who provided the illustrations in Chapter Two.

Finally we are indebted to our publisher, Appleton-Century-Crofts and especially to their executive medical editor, Doreen Berne, who supervised the project, Jody Thum, the production editor, and Jean Sabato, the art director.

Computed Tomography of the Eye and Orbit

CHAPTER ONE

Anatomy
Discussion

THE BONY ORBIT

The orbital cavities are located in a parasagittal plane of the skull between the facial skeleton and cranium. Each orbit is roughly pyramidal in shape, with seven bones contributing to the walls: frontal, maxilla, sphenoid, zygoma, ethmoid, lacrimal, and palatine. Above each orbit is the anterior cranial fossa; medially, the ethmoid sinus; below, the maxillary sinus; posteromedially, the middle cranial fossa, and posterolaterally, the temporal fossa. The medial walls of the orbits are almost parallel, whereas the lateral walls subtend an angle of approximately 90° with each other. The orbital roof is formed largely by the orbital plate of the frontal bone anteriorly, with a smaller contribution posteriorly by the lesser wing of the sphenoid. The medial wall is formed mainly by the orbital plate of the ethmoid, with a contribution anteriorly by the lacrimal bone and posteriorly by the body of the sphenoid. The ethmoid plate (lamina papyryacea) separating the orbit from the ethmoid air cells is very thin and is perforated by small foramina allowing vascular communications. The orbital floor is formed mainly by the orbital plate of the maxilla, with lesser contributions by the orbital surface of the zygomatic bone anterolaterally and the orbital process of the palatine bone at the apex. The infraorbital groove runs forward from about the middle of the inferior orbital fissure and soon becomes roofed over as the infraorbital canal. The lateral orbital wall is formed by the greater wing of the sphenoid posteriorly and the zygomatic bone anteriorly. The sphenoidal portion of the lateral wall is separated from the roof by the superior orbital fissure and from the floor by the inferior orbital fissure. The lateral wall separates the orbit anteriorly from the temporal fossa containing the temporalis muscle and posteriorly from the middle cranial fossa and middle lobe of the brain. The superior orbital fissure separates the greater and lesser wings of the sphenoid and lies between the roof and the lateral wall of the orbit. It is separated from the optic canal at its medial aspect by the posterior root of the lesser wing of the sphenoid.

THE OPTIC CANAL

The optic canal provides a communication between the middle cranial fossa and orbital apex. The canal is formed by the two roots of the lesser sphenoid wing and is directed anteriorly, laterally, and inferiorly, the axis forming an angle of approximately 37° with the midsagittal plane and 30° with Reid's baseline.[1] The canal is roughly cylindrical and is funneled in one plane at both ends, i.e., the intracranial end of the canal is oval with its long axis horizontal, whereas the orbital end of the canal is oval with the long axis vertical. The midportion of the canal is round. The measurements are: orbital end, 5 × 6 mm; middle, 5 × 5 mm; and intracranial end, 4.5 × 6 mm. The roof of the canal is 8 to 10 mm long, whereas the floor and lateral walls are 6 to 8 mm long. The medial wall of the optic canal is rather regularly adjacent to the sphenoid sinus, occasionally actually projecting into it.[2] The optic canal transmits the optic nerve and its coverings of dura, arachnoid, and pia. The ophthalmic artery lies below and is embedded in the dural sheath. Sympathetic nerve branches accompany the artery. The ophthalmic artery crosses below the nerve from medial at the posterior end of the canal to exit inferolaterally to the nerve at the orbital end. The pia forms a sheath closely adherent to the nerve. The dura serves as a periosteal lining of the canal and splits at the orbital end to become continuous with the periobita, as well as continuing as the dural sheath of the intraorbital optic nerve.

THE OPTIC NERVE

Developmentally, the optic nerve is a fiber tract joining two portions of the brain,[3] its fibers containing glial and not Schwann cells, and it is surrounded by meninges, unlike any peripheral nerves. The total length of the optic nerve is about 4 to 5 cm, and it has four sections: an intracranial prechiasmal part, about 10 mm in length; an intracanalicular part 6 mm in length; an intraorbital part of about 25 to 30 mm (which has a slightly sinuous course, with the length of the optic nerve being about 6 mm greater than the distance from the optic canal to the ocular bulb); and intraocular section, where the optic nerve penetrates the sclera, measuring approximately 0.7 to 1.5 mm in length. The intraorbital optic nerve is enclosed in three sheaths that are continuous with the membranes of the brain and extend along the optic nerve up to the eyeball. The outer sheath, derived from the dura mater is thick and fibrous and blends anteriorly with the sclera. Posteriorly, at the optic canal, it splits to blend with the periosteum of the optic canal and the periosteum (periorbita) of the orbit. The fibrous annulus of Zinn, formed by the convergence of the origins of the rectus muscles, also fuses to the dura of the optic nerve at the optic canal. The intermediate sheath of the optic nerve is derived from the arachnoid mater and is thin and delicate. The subarachnoid space is continuous with the intracranial subarachnoid space, and cerebrospinal fluid (CSF) surrounds the optic nerve up to the lamina cribrosa (papilla) of the eye ball.[4] The inner sheath derived from pia is vascular and invests the nerve. From its deep surface, septa pass into the nerve and subdivide it into bundles.

THE OPTIC CHIASM

The optic chiasm is a flattened quadrilateral bundle of nerve fibers situated at the junction of the anterior wall and the floor of the third ventricle, forming the floor of the chiasmatic recess. It measures about 12 mm in transverse diameter and about 8 mm in sagittal diameter. Anterolaterally it is continuous with the intracranial optic nerves, and posterolaterally with the optic tracts. It lies obliquely, with the posterior border higher than the anterior border, suspended and surrounded by CSF.

ORBITAL VESSELS

Ophthalmic Artery

The ophthalmic artery arises intracranially from the medial side of the internal carotid artery just after this vessel has traversed the cavernous sinus and pierced the dura. Within the optic canal the ophthalmic artery lies inferolateral to the optic nerve contained with the dural sheath of the nerve. It enters the orbit in the muscle cone running inferolateral to the optic nerve for a short distance but soon crosses over the nerve between the nerve and superior rectus muscle (in 15 percent it crosses beneath the nerve) and continues anteriorly to reach the medial orbital wall. Further forward, it lies between the medial rectus and superior oblique muscles up to the maxillary process of the frontal bone. Beyond the orbit the ophthalmic artery supplies the forehead and lateral wall of the nose. Within the orbit it gives off a number of variable branches, about 14 in number,[3] the most important of which is the central retinal artery. Other branches include the ciliary, ethmoidal, lacrimal, muscular, and supratrochlear arteries.

Orbital Veins

The orbital venous drainage occurs mostly via a superior ophthalmic vein and to a lesser extent by an inferior ophthalmic vein. These are tortuous, with many plexiform anastomoses, and like most facial veins they are valveless. The superior ophthalmic vein is formed near the root of the nose by anastomosis of the angular, nasofrontal, and supraorbital veins. It then travels posterolaterally through the orbit, penetrating the muscle cone in midorbit. It then runs deep to the superior rectus muscle and leaves the orbit near the annulus of Zinn via the superior orbital fissure and drains into the cavernous sinus. The inferior ophthalmic vein commences as a plexus near the front of the orbit and extends posteriorly on the inferior rectus, communicating with the superior ophthalmic vein and draining into the pterygoid plexus via the inferior orbital fissure.

Lymphatics

The orbit contains no lymphatic capillaries or lymphoid tissue. The eyelids, conjunctiva, and lacrimal glands do contain a lymphatic system.

EXTRAOCULAR MUSCLES

There are six extrinsic (striated) muscles that move the ocular globe: superior, inferior, medial, and lateral rectus; and superior and inferior oblique muscles. An additional muscle, the levator palpebrae superioris, arises from the lesser wing of the sphenoid, passes forward immediately above the superior rectus, and inserts into the upper eyelid. The sheath of the levator attaches below to that of the superior rectus. The four rectus muscles have a common origin at the apex in the annulus of Zinn, which is a short tendinous ring encircling the optic foramen and medial end of the superior orbital fissure. The muscle extends forwards as separate bundles but is joined together by an intermuscular fascial membrane, providing an inner or intraconal space and an extraconal or peripheral space. Each rectus muscle inserts separately into the sclera of the globe. The superior oblique is the longest and thinnest eye muscle. It arises superomedially to the optic foramen and passes anteriorly between the roof and medial wall to the trochlea. About 1 cm posterior to the trochlea, the muscle is replaced by a rounded tendon that passes through the pulley, turning sharply medially to insert into the globe below the superior rectus. The trochlea consists of a U-shaped piece of fibrocartilage. The inferior oblique is the only extrinsic muscle to take origin from the front of the orbit, arising on the orbital plate of the maxilla just lateral to the orifice of the nasolacrimal duct. It passes laterally and posteriorly (roughly parallel with the tendon of the superior oblique) between the inferior rectus and the orbital floor to insert in the posterolateral aspect of the globe.

ORBITAL FASCIA

There are several components to the orbital fascia.

Tenon's Capsule
Tenon's capsule (the fascia bulbi) is a thin fibrous membrane that envelops the globe from the margin of the cornea to the optic nerve. It is separated from the sclera, providing a potential space—the episcleral space. This space is traversed by delicate bands of connective tissue that extend between the sclera and fascia[5] and can be involved in inflammatory conditions. Tenon's capsule is related by various reflections to the aponeuroses and check ligaments of the extraocular muscles, conjunctiva, and globe. This network of interconnections facilitates the extension of tenonitis to the orbital tissues.[6] The intermuscular fascial membrane and trabeculae of the orbital fat are part of this extensive fascial connective tissue system of the globe and orbit.

Intermuscular Membrane
The intermuscular membrane is an aponeurotic sheath derived from the sheaths of the four rectus muscles. In some individuals it may be a poorly defined structure.[7] Together with the rectus muscles, it separates the intra- and extraconal spaces.

Orbital Septum
The orbital septum is a thin connective tissue membrane that attaches around the orbital margin, where it is continuous with the periosteum. This circumferential structure extends centrally to become attached to the tarsal plates of the eyelids. It is perforated by vessels and nerves that pass from the orbital cavity to the face and scalp, by the palpebral part of the lacrimal gland, and by the aponeurosis of the levator palpebrae superioris.[5] The soft-tissue space anterior to the orbital septum is the preseptal space. The soft tissues confined within the periorbita deep to the orbital septum constitutes the orbit proper. The orbital septum is an important barrier to the spread of preseptal or eyelid inflammation to the posterior compartment.

ORBITAL FAT

The orbital contents are invested by adipose tissue subdivided into lobules by fine fibrous septa. The orbital fat extends from the apex to the orbital septum anteriorly, sometimes bulging it forwards as it slackens with age. The consistency of the fat and the amount of connective tissue between the fat lobules vary in different parts of the orbit. The intermuscular membrane separates the fat into a central or intramuscular portion and a peripheral fat compartment. The central fat is loose, allowing for movements of the optic nerve; and is finely lobulated with thin septa. At the back of the globe the septa insert into Tenon's capsule. The peripheral fat is situated between the rectus muscles and the periorbita, and limited anteriorly by the septum. The peripheral layer of fat is subdivided into four discreet lobules[3] situated mainly in the intermuscular spaces.

LACRIMAL GLAND

The lacrimal gland is about the size of an almond and occupies the lacrimal gland fossa on the medial surface of the zygomatic process of the frontal bone, extending down almost to the lateral angle of the globe. The gland is divided into a larger upper or orbital lobe and a smaller lower or palpebral lobe. The two lobes are separated from each other by the expanded insertion of the levator palpebrae superioris.

COMPUTED TOMOGRAPHIC (CT) MANIFESTATIONS

By virtue of the large amount of orbital fat surrounding the various components of the orbit, visualization of the small structures is exceptional. In different CT planes, the extraocular muscles, vessels, and nerves can be clearly identified. However, the delineation of these structures in their part or whole depends on several factors, including section thickness, angle of the plane of scan relative to the orbit, and the resolution of the scanner. For example, an early-generation CT scanner resolving only 3.5 line pairs/cm could identify the ophthalmic artery in less than 1 percent of the cases, whereas a new high-resolution scanner resolving 10 line pairs/cm could identify this artery in all cases.[8] The orbital fat has a CT value of approximately −100 Hounsfield (H) units. Without contrast enhancement, the arteries, veins, nerves, and muscles of the orbit measure 30 to 35 H units, providing a difference of about 130 H units. Because of this large difference in absorption values without contrast material, utilization of contrast enhancement does not significantly increase visualization of these structures. Detail is dependent on spatial rather than added contrast resolution.[8]

REFERENCES

1. Goalwin HA: The precise roentgenography and measurement of the optic canal. AJR 13:480–484, 1925

2. Van Alyea OE: Sphenoid sinus: Anatomic study with consideration of the clinical significance of the structural characteristics of the sphenoid sinus. Arch Otolaryngol 34:225–253, 1941

3. Wolff E: Anatomy of the Eye and Orbit, 7th ed. Philadelphia, Saunders, 1976

4. Whitnall SE: Anatomy of the Human Orbit and Accessory Organs of Vision, 4th ed. London, Oxford University Press, 1932

5. Williams PL, Warwick R: Functional Neuroanatomy of Man. Philadelphia, Saunders, 1975, p 1128

6. Jones IS, Jakobiec FA: Diseases of the Orbit. Hagerstown, Md., Harper & Row, 1979

7. Poirier P: Traite d'Anatomie Humaine, 3rd ed, Vol 5, fasc 2: Les Organes du Sens, Paris, Maisson, 1911

8. Weinstein MA, Modic MT, Risius B, et al: Visualization of the arteries, veins, and nerves of the orbit by sector computed tomography. Radiology 138:83–87, 1981

Illustrations

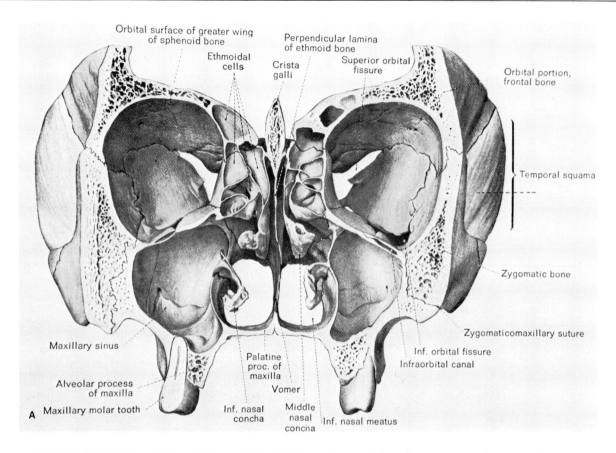

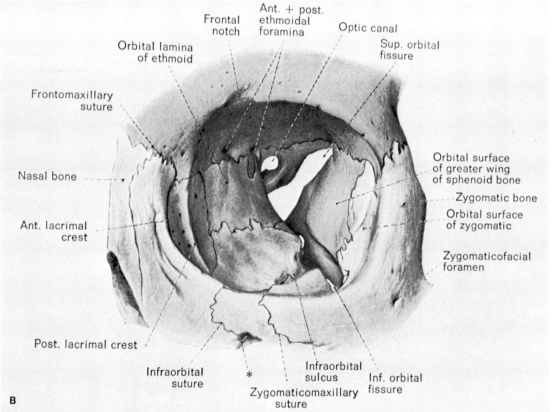

Figure 1.A. Coronal section through orbits. **B.** Apical view of orbit, demonstrating bony relationships.*

Reprinted from Sobotta J, Figge FHJ: Atlas of Human Anatomy. Baltimore, Urban and Schwarzenberg, 1977, Vol 1, p 61, with permission.

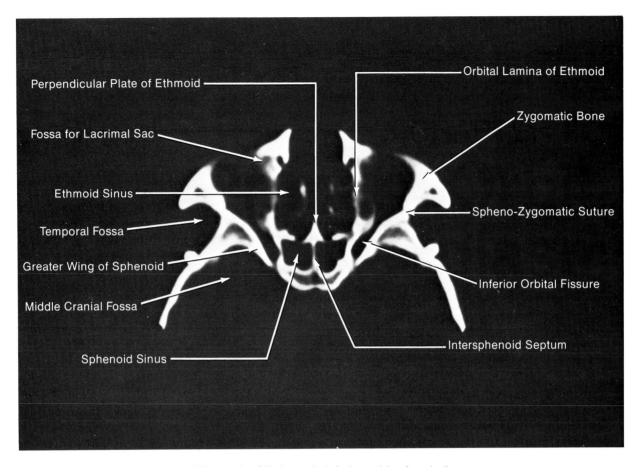

Figure 2. CT through inferior orbit of a skull.

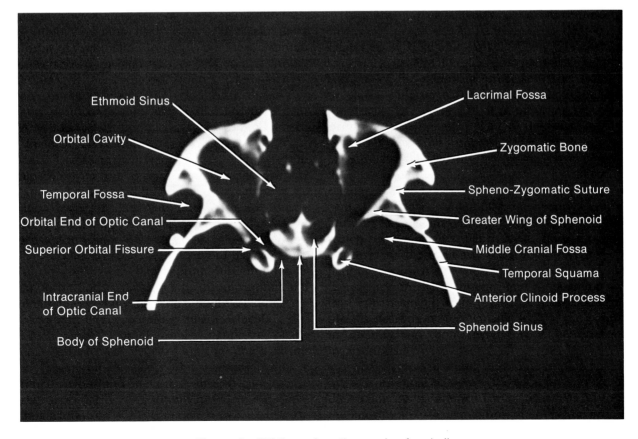

Figure 3. CT through optic canals of a skull.

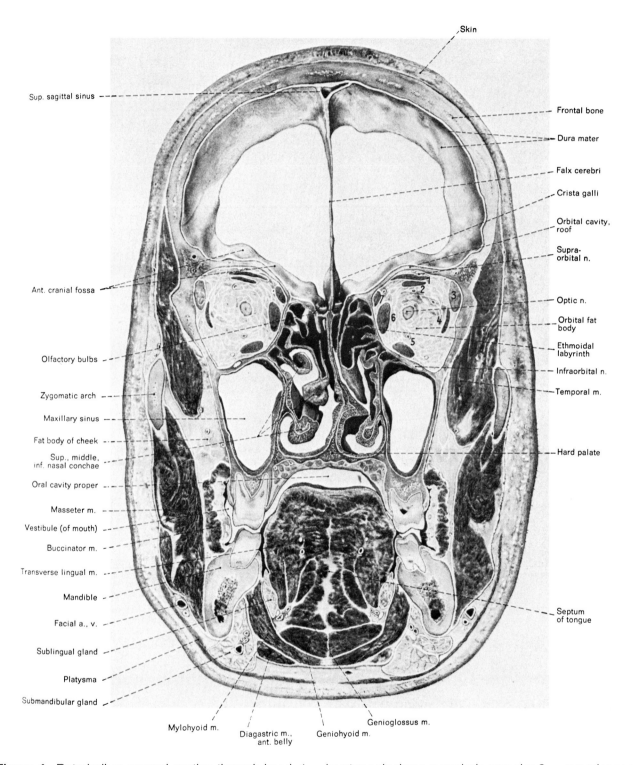

Figure 4. Retrobulbar coronal section through head. 1 = levator palpebrae superioris muscle; 2 = superior rectus; 3 = lacrimal gland; 4 = lateral rectus; 5 = inferior rectus. 6 = medial rectus; 7 = superior oblique.*

Reprinted from Sobotta J, Figge FHJ: Atlas of Human Anatomy. Baltimore, Urban and Schwarzenberg, 1977, Vol 2, p 149, with permission.

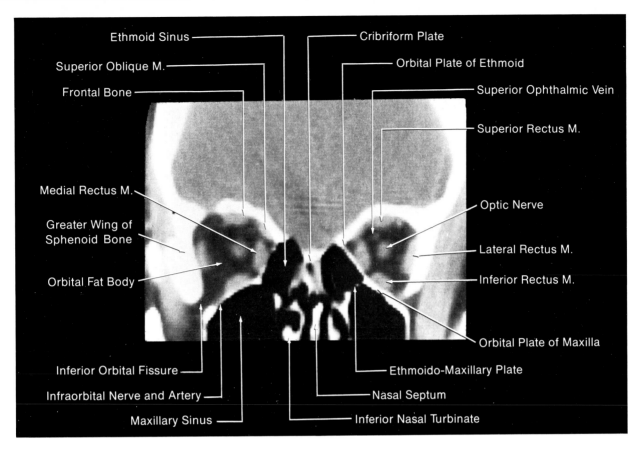

Figure 5. Coronal CT through retrobulbar area.

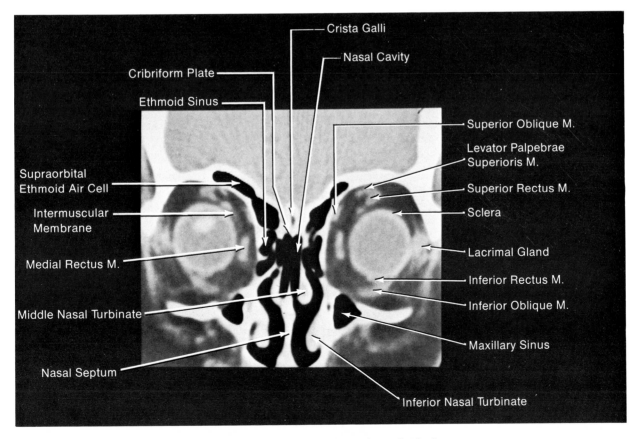

Figure 6. Coronal CT through ocular bulbs.

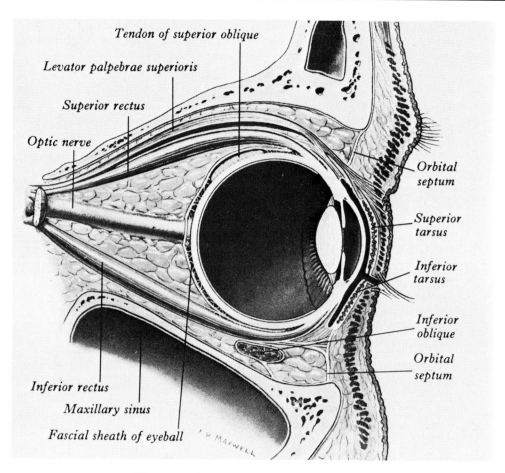

Figure 7. Sagittal section through orbit.*

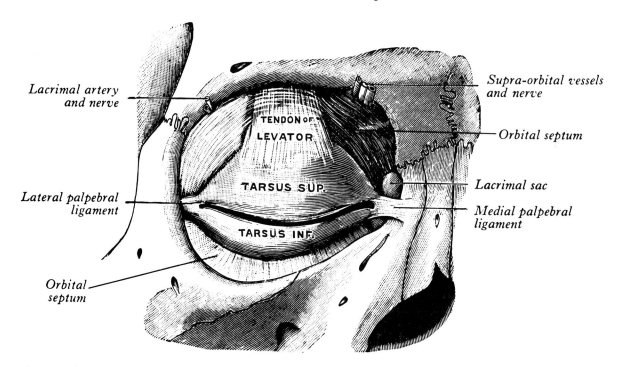

Figure 8. Anterior aspect of the tarsi and their ligaments. The orbital septum separates the preseptal or periorbital compartment from the orbit proper.*

*Reprinted from Williams PL, Warwick R: *Functional Neuroanatomy of Man*, ed 35. Edinburgh, Scotland, Churchill Livingstone, 1975, pp 1123, 1131, with permission.*

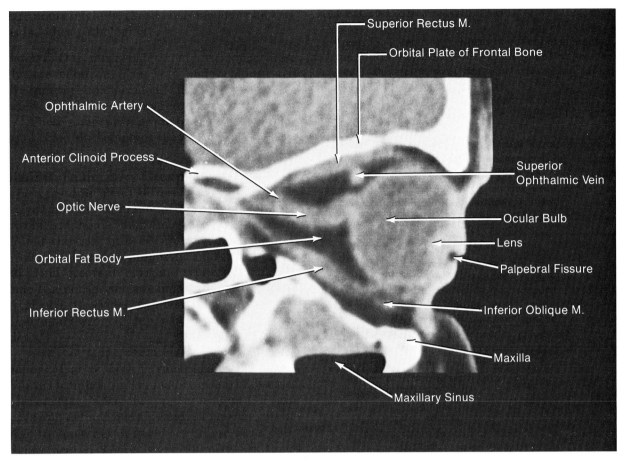

Figure 9. Sagittal CT through a cadaver orbit. Fluid accumulation in antral roof is due to vertex down position.

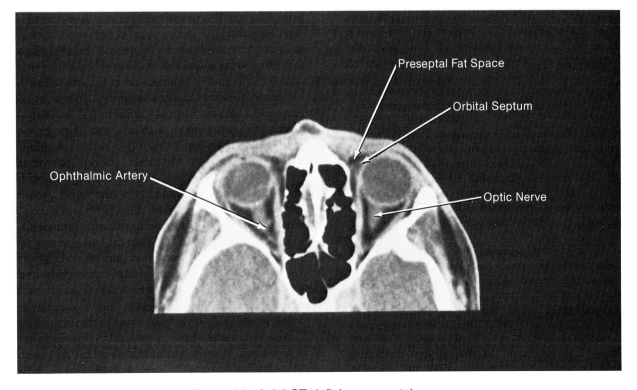

Figure 10. Axial CT defining preseptal space.

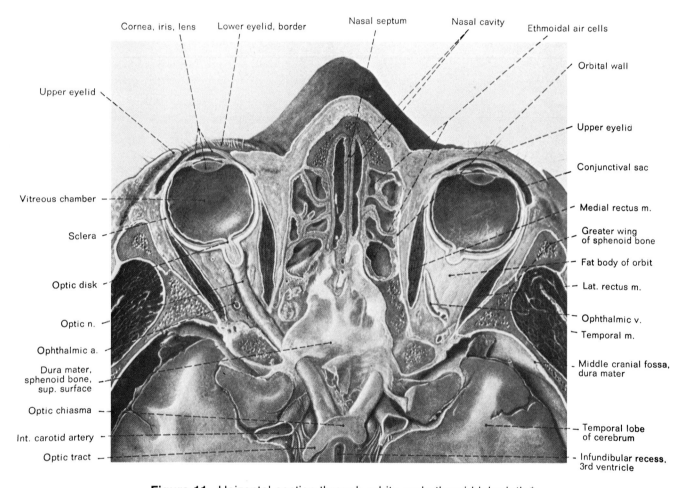

Figure 11. Hoizontal section through orbits and ethmoid labyrinth.*

Reprinted from Sobotta J, Figge FHJ: Atlas of Human Anatomy. Baltimore, Urban and Schwarzenberg, 1977, Vol 2, p 151, with permission.

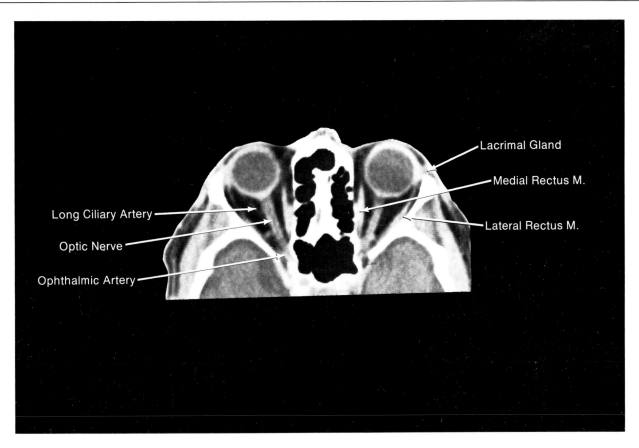

Figure 12. Detail of the optic nerve. The central linear lucency represents the optic nerve surrounded by a denser optic nerve sheath.

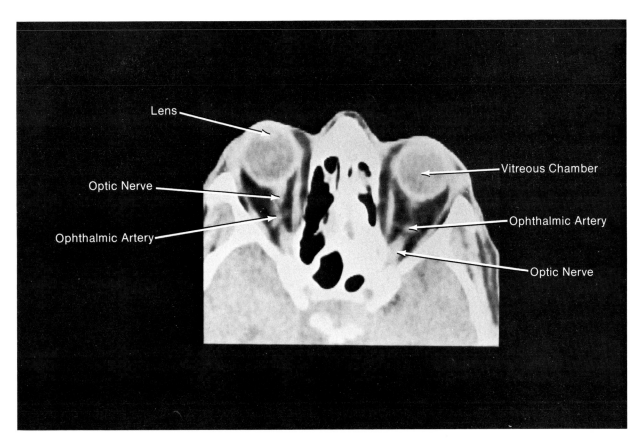

Figure 13. Ophthalmic artery crosses over the optic nerve.

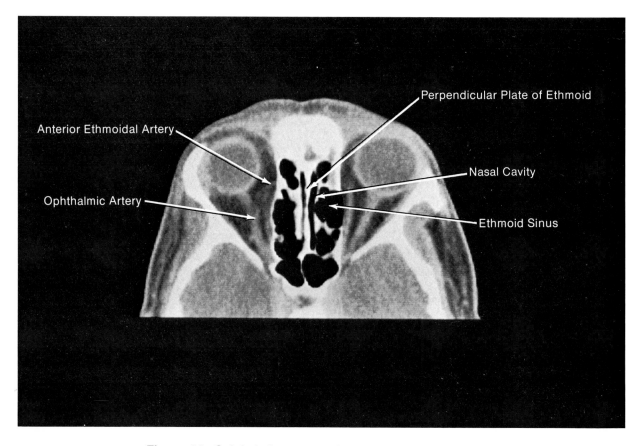

Figure 14. Ophthalmic artery and anterior ethmoidal branch.

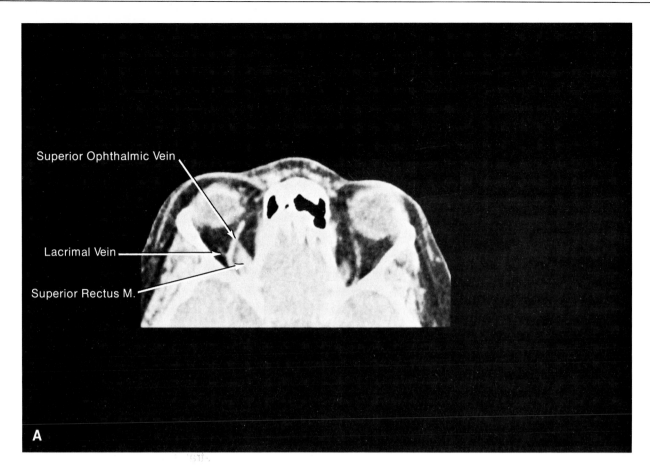

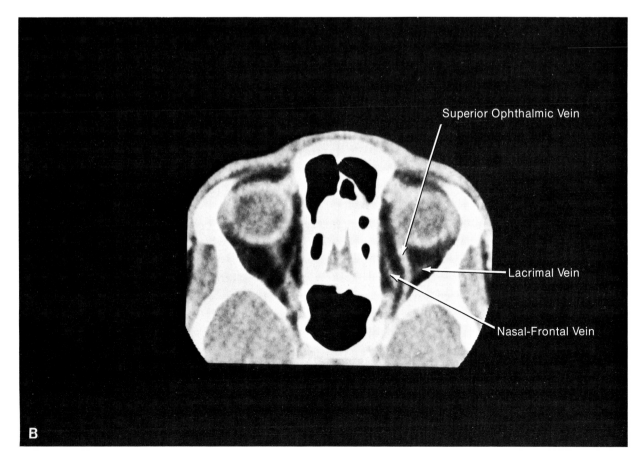

Figure 15. A and B. Venous anatomy. The superior ophthalmic vein crosses deep to the superior rectus muscle.

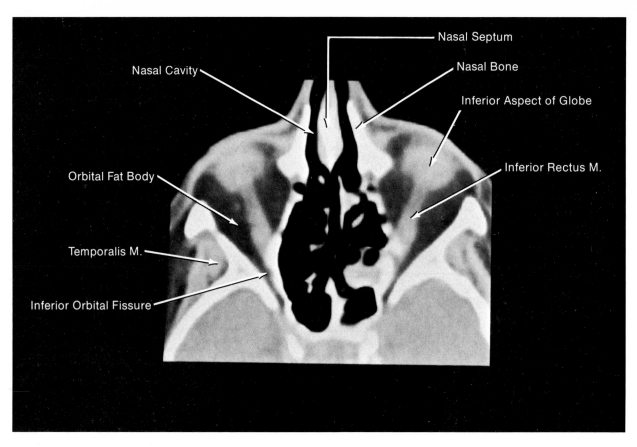

Figure 16. Inferior orbital section with CT axis parallel to orbital floor demonstrates the inferior rectus muscle in its entirety.

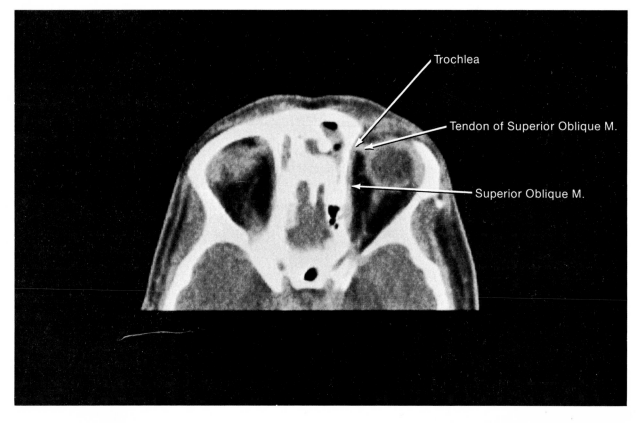

Figure 17. Upper orbital section demonstrates the superior oblique muscle.

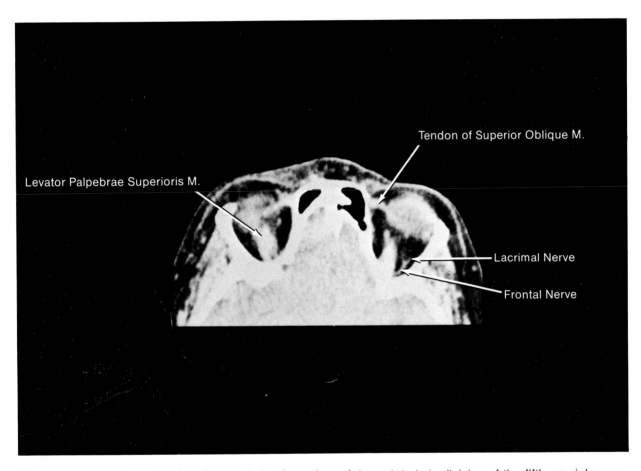

Figure 18. High orbital section demonstrates branches of the ophthalmic division of the fifth cranial nerve.

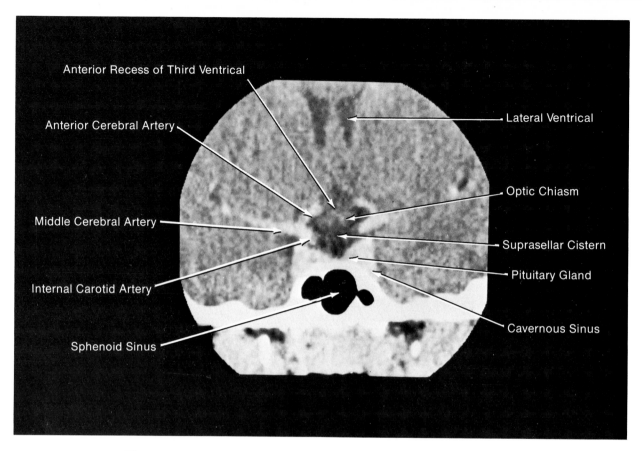

Figure 19. Contrast-enhanced coronal CT through the optic chiasm.

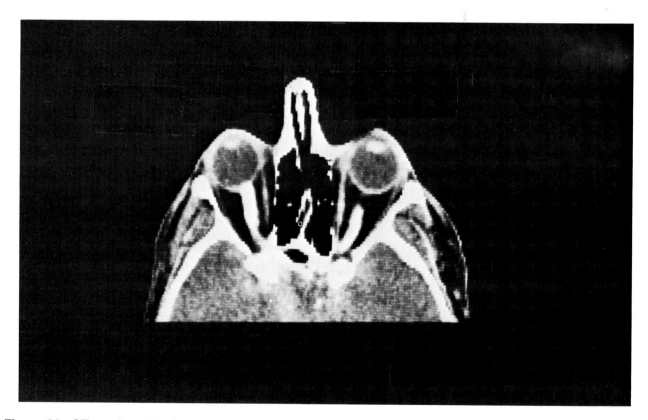

Figure 20. CT metrizamide cisternogram with contrast outlining both optic nerves. The perioptic subarachnoid space communicates with the basal cisterns.

CHAPTER TWO

Technique

The anterior visual pathways and their related orbital structures present a unique challenge to the conscientious computed tomographer. The cone-shaped orbit contains a mobile ocular globe attached to diverging extraocular muscles. The intraorbital optic nerve has a serpiginous configuration that changes its axis as it penetrates the optic canal to become the optic chiasm. Thus, it can be stated that there is no single optimal plane of section for CT scanning of the orbit and anterior visual pathways.

For orientation, it is important to identify some skeletal and radiographic landmarks. The anthropologic baseline (Reid's baseline or the Frankfurt-Virchow line) is a line extending from the inferior orbital rim to the upper margin of the external auditory meatus. The plane of the optic canal subtends an angle of $-30°$ with Reid's baseline and $-20°$ with the orbitomeatal line[1-3] (Fig. 2.C).

From early in the CT experience, it was established that scanning the orbit in a plane parallel to Reid's baseline provided satisfactory images.[4] In the primary position of gaze, however, the intraorbital optic nerve is tortuous in a vertical plane, with the central part of the nerve situated more caudal than the proximal and distal parts[5] (Fig. 1.A). Any single CT slice will always section the optic nerve obliquely (Fig. 1.B). The image of the optic nerve depends on the slice thickness.[6] Thick sections (8 to 10 mm) result in volume-averaging with orbital fat but will include the entire thickness of the optic nerve, producing a uniformly dense optic nerve. In view of the reduced spatial resolution with thick sections, however, 8- to 10-mm sections are not recommended. At the other extreme, 1.5- to 2-mm sec-

tions produce high-quality images, but such exquisite detail is not routinely required. These very thin slices, however, can section the optic nerve in a plane extending through its entire length, albeit obliquely. The result is an optic nerve of uniform density.

Slice thickness of approximately 5 mm is optimal for most orbital scanning, providing adequate resolution of the small structures. In the primary position of gaze, a 5-mm section in a plane parallel to Reid's baseline will incur volume-averaging with orbital fat in the midpoint of the optic nerve as it dips caudally (Fig. 1). This produces a tapered configuration to the central part of the nerve or, in more extreme cases, a central hypodensity.[5]

Gaze shifts can alter the configuration of the optic nerve quite considerably. With extreme upward gaze, as the anterior part of the globe rotates upward, the optic nerve is displaced downwards with the posterior globe. This tends to straighten out most of the optic nerve except the most anterior part, where it curves upward to attach to the globe (Fig. 2.A). This maneuver can be used to advantage during scanning. If the orbit is now scanned in a plane approximating that of the orbital floor, the section will include most of the optic nerve along its axis[7] (Fig. 2.B). Only the most anterior part of the nerve will not be encompassed in this section, but is obtained on the next cranial section. It turns out that this plane of section is also the most optimal for the optic canal (Fig. 2.C).

As stated previously, the optic canal subtends an angle of $-30°$ with Reid's baseline (Fig. 2.C). This is well known to all radiologists who recognize the optic canal seen en face in the outer lower quadrant of the

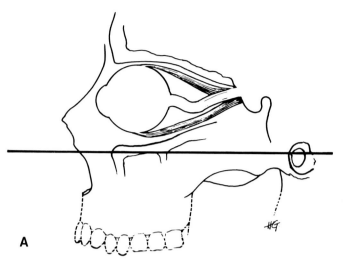

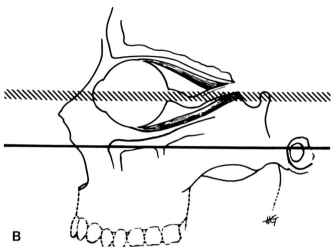

Figure 1.A. Sagittal view through orbit. Reid's baseline extends from the inferior orbital rim to the external auditory meatus. In the primary position of gaze, there is a sagittal tortuosity to the optic nerve with the central part of the nerve convex downwards.

Figure 1.B. The crosshatched line represents a 5-mm CT section parallel to Reid's baseline. The posterior aspect of the nerve is sectioned obliquely. Partial voluming of the central part of the nerve with orbital fat is apparent.

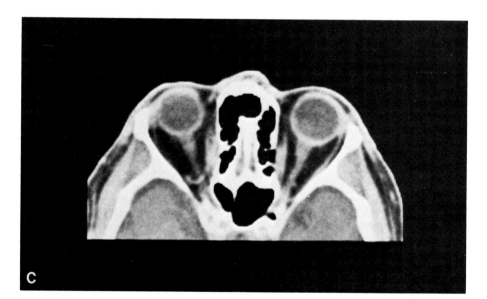

Figure 1.C. CT corresponding to B. Due to volume-averaging with orbital fat, the central part of the optic nerves has a tapered configuration.

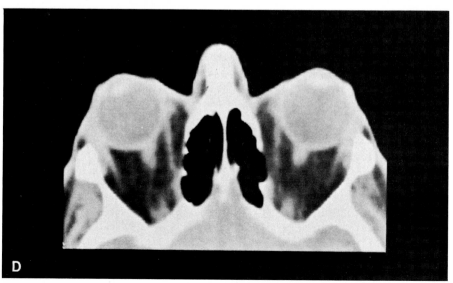

Figure 1.D. More marked volume-averaging than in C, resulting in central hypodensities involving both optic nerves.

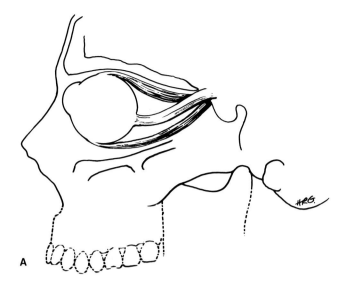

Figure 2.A. Sagittal view of orbit, with eye in extreme upgaze position. As the posterior globe moves inferiorly, the optic nerve moves downwards and straightens out in the lower orbit.

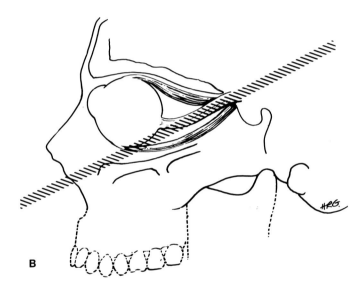

Figure 2.B. The crosshatched lines represent a CT section angled downwards approximately −30° to Reid's baseline. With the eye in the extreme upgaze position, most of the optic nerve will be included in this CT section. Only the most anterior part of the nerve extends out of the plane of section.

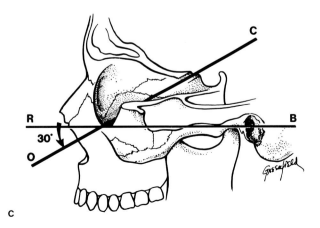

Figure 2.C. Lateral view of the orbit exposing the optic canal. Line OC extends through the axis of the optic canal and subtends an angle of −30°, with line RB representing Reid's baseline. Line OC is in the same plane as the CT section represented in B.

continued

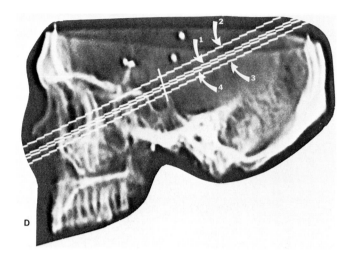

Figure 2.D. Lateral digital skull radiograph. Electronically generated line 1 extends from the tuberculum sella to a point just above the inferior orbital rim. This corresponds to line OC in C. Scans 2 and 3 are 5-mm craniad and caudad, respectively, to 1. Scan 4 is 1-mm caudad to scan 1.*

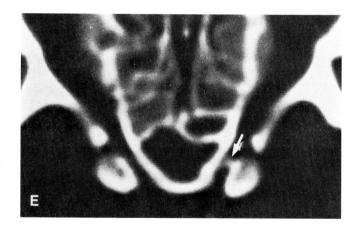

Figure 2.E. CT of optic canals corresponding to scan 1 in D. The section is perfectly aligned with axis of the right optic canal, but due to slight rotation, bone at the orbital end of the left optic canal (arrow) is included.*

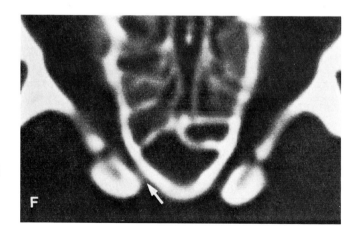

Figure 2.F. CT of optic canals corresponding to scan 4 in D. The section is now perfectly aligned with the axis of the left optic canal. Bone at the intracranial end of the right optic canal (arrow) is included.*

*Reprinted from Hammerschlag SB, O'Reilly GV, Naheedy MH: Computed tomography of the optic canals. AJNR 2:594, © 1981, with permission.

orbit in the conventional optic foramen view. The optic canal should be scanned in a section that is parallel to its axis, i.e., −30° to Reid's baseline. What follows is a simple and rapid method of imaging the orbit, optic nerve, and optic canal in an axial plane. This method focuses maximally on the optic nerve and canal, but adequate detail of the remainder of the structures—including the extraocular muscles, orbital apex, and bony margins—is also obtained.

OPTIMAL METHOD FOR AXIAL ORBITAL SCANNING

With the patient supine, the head is placed in a slightly hyperextended position. A lateral-view digital radiograph is obtained. The electronically generated localizer line to indicate the angle of scan is adjusted so that the plane of scan extends from the tip of the anterior clinoids to a point slightly craniad to the inferior orbital rim. If the anterior clinoids cannot be identified, the tuberculum sella will suffice. This line corresponds to the axis of the optic canal and subtends an angle of −30° to Reid's baseline.[3] A few degrees of gantry tilt are usually necessary to achieve precise alignment with the angle of the localizer line on the digital radiograph. The first scan should be placed 5-mm caudade to the localizer line so as to include the most inferior orbital structures. The inferior rectus muscle is often imaged along its axis (see Chap. 1, Fig. 16). A series of about six contiguous 5-mm scans without overlap is obtained. It may be necessary to obtain one or two additional scans inbetween the original slices, so as to precisely section through the axis of the optic canal without including the bony margins of the floor or the roof of the canal (Fig. 2D–F). As the vertical height of the central part of the canal is about 5 mm, thicker sections will result in volume-averaging with bone.

Prior to initiating each scan, the patient is instructed to look upwards, thus positioning the globe in the upward gaze configuration. The optic nerve is thereby straightened with its axis in the same plane as the optic canal (Fig. 3). Most adult patients can maintain the upward gaze position for the duration of each scan without difficulty. The approach is modified slightly for children, in whom there is less angulation of the optic canal than in adults.[8] In infancy, about 10° less angulation, i.e., −20° to Reid's baseline, is required, with increasing angulation until the −30° of the adult configuration is reached in adolescence. There is no control of gaze shifts in infants and young children, but visualization of the optic nerve is usually adequate.

The optic canal cannot be accurately delineated unless the CT section is precisely through its axis. Therefore, a scan with an angle that is significantly less than the required −30° to Reid's baseline will section the canal obliquely and give it a spurious funneled configuration (Fig. 4).

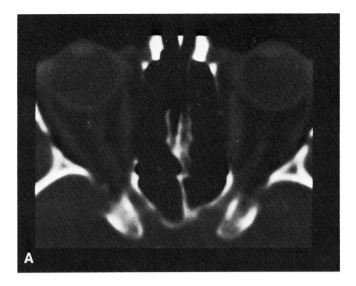

Figure 3.A. Scan through the axis of the optic canals with bone settings in a normal patient. Symmetrical flaring of the intracranial aspect of both optic canals is a normal variant.*

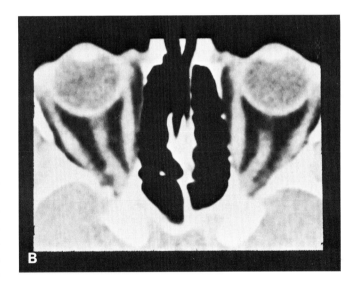

Figure 3.B. Same image as in A, with soft-tissue settings. The patient was instructed to fixate in upgaze during scanning. Visualization of most of the intraorbital optic nerves is satisfactory. Only the most anterior part of the nerves are not completely imaged.*

*Reprinted from Hammerschlag SB, O'Reilly GV, Naheedy MH: Computed tomography of the optic canals. AJNR 2:594, © 1981, with permission.

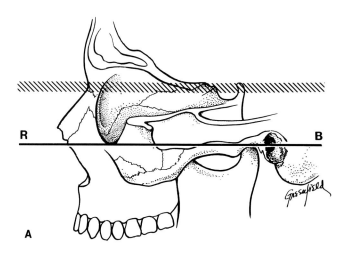

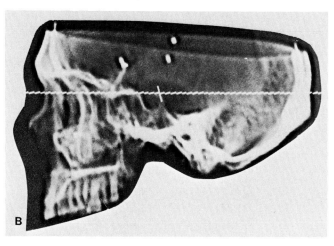

Figure 4.A. Lateral view of orbit with optic canal exposed. The crosshatched area represents a 5-mm CT section extending through the optic canals, in a plane parallel to line RB representing Reid's baseline. The optic canals are sectioned obliquely.

Figure 4.B. Lateral digital skull radiograph. The localizer line indicates a section through the optic canal in a plane parallel to Reid's baseline, corresponding to the crosshatched line in A.*

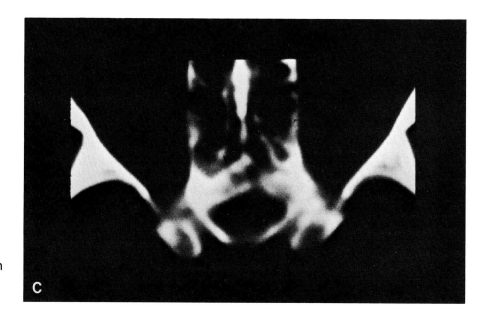

Figure 4.C. CT of optic canals corresponding to B. There is spurious funneling of the optic canals due to the oblique plane of section through the cylindrically shaped optic canals.*

THE OPTIC CHIASM

To complete the examination of the anterior visual pathways, the intracranial optic nerves and optic chiasm should be imaged. This requires a change of angulation, preferably obtained by means of the lateral digital radiograph and localizer line. The chiasm is imaged optimally in a plane parallel to Reid's baseline, scanning through the suprasellar region[9] (Fig. 4B). Contrast material should be given to detect abnormal enhancement, as well as to delineate the normal adjacent vascular structures such as the carotid arteries and in-

fundibulum. If this initial survey through the suprasellar region reveals no pathologic features, but the degree of suspicion for abnormality remains high, further studies of the optic chiasm are justified. First, both axial and direct coronal scans (parallel and perpendicular to Reid's baseline), using very thin sections (preferably 1.5 to 2 mm, or at most 4 to 5 mm) and IV contrast administration may detect a subtle abnormality. The most sensitive examination, however, is a CT metrizamide cisternogram using very thin sections in either the axial or coronal plane, or both.[9,10] This investigation should be undertaken without reluctance if there is any question of a chiasmatic-related lesion that has not been adequately delineated on prior studies. This procedure entails a high lumbar puncture with intrathecal injection of 4 to 5 ml metrizamide (170 mg I/ml). With the patient in the prone position, the table is tilted down about 40° for two minutes and then returned to the horizontal position and transported to the CT scanner for imaging as described above. The patient should remain prone until transferred to the scanning table.

The above method describes the optimal approach for scanning to delineate structures related primarily to vision loss. Most orbital scanning, however, is performed to demonstrate a cause for exophthalmos. In these instances, precise visualization of the optic canal is usually not crucial, and it is therefore acceptable to scan the orbit in a plane parallel to Reid's baseline with the patient maintaining the primary position of gaze. Regardless of gaze manipulation during scanning, complete delineation of the optic nerve in such cases is often not possible because of displacement by the underlying mass. We have found, however, that to avoid confusion, it is as well to standardize the orbital CT technique, and we therefore scan all orbits regardless of symptomatology in the −30° to Reid's baseline.

Other points needing further elaboration are the use of IV contrast, supplementary projections, evaluation of the extraocular muscles, and radiation dosimetry.

CONTRAST ENHANCEMENT

As was outlined in Chapter 1 (under CT Manifestations), IV contrast administration does not significantly increase visualization of the normal intraorbital structures. The definition of a pathologic lesion is often increased with contrast enhancement, but generally this adds little specificity. Therefore, contrast administration for intraorbital pathology is not mandatory, and is not routinely given. There are, however, two exceptions. Intravenous contrast should always be given when evaluating the optic chiasm and perisellar region (30 to 40 g I adult dose infused over five minutes, starting while the patient is being positioned). The slight or moderate enhancement of a small optic chiasm glioma may be enough to detect a subtle abnormality and at least influence the decision to proceed with the more definitive CT metrizamide cisternogram. Contrast should also be given in any case where there is a suspicion of a combined intraorbital-intracranial lesion. The intracranial component may only be revealed with enhancement. Therefore, detection of any abnormality of the bony margins of the orbit bordering the intracranial compartment or the temporal fossa should be followed with a contrast study. The same, however, does not apply to a combined sinus-orbit lesion, in which contrast enhancement provides little additional information. The utilization of contrast enhancement

in separating orbital abscess from orbital cellulitis has been helpful in some cases, but its role has not yet been fully determined.

CORONAL AND SAGITTAL PROJECTIONS

Although thin-section (5-mm) axial scanning will detect most abnormalities within the orbit, because of the close proximity of the structures—specifically at the orbital apex and the extraconal space between the muscle cone and the bony margins—it becomes important to obtain a vertical perspective to fully appreciate these relationships. This is achieved by coronal imaging incorporated as part of the routine of the orbital CT study. Sagittal views are helpful, but much less so than coronal views: however, in cases of trauma to the orbital floor, sagittal perspective is essential.[11]

Coronal and sagittal views can be obtained directly by head and gantry manipulation.[12–17] Alternatively, with the newer generation of CT scanners these can be obtained by means of contiguous or overlapping thin axial sections with data manipulation that permits multiplanar reformations.[18–20]

Therefore, as a general principle, coronal images should routinely supplement the axial study. Forgoing this additional projection may result in an incomplete evaluation. Extraocular muscle thickening, particularly involving the inferior rectus, can be missed. Conversely, extraocular muscle thickening can mimic an apical mass on axial views alone[21,22] (Fig. 5). Apparent apical masses can result from inadvertent oblique sectioning of the normal muscle cone (Fig. 6). This may occur if the angle of section parallels or is greater than the plane of the orbital roof, as is typically used for brain CT. Again, supplementary coronal views would resolve any questions.

It is also readily apparent that a vertical perspective to the orbit is helpful in foreign-body localization, as well as in the surgical planning for any orbital mass. Sagittal views along the axis of the inferior rectus muscle have a special application in orbital floor blowout fractures, where they are necessary to determine the precise relationship of the inferior rectus muscle to the defect in the floor. Coronal views alone are inadequate to make this determination.[11]

Coronal views can be obtained by either direct scanning or computer reformations. Direct coronal CT can be performed with the patient positioned prone or supine.[23] Disadvantages of this technique are that it is uncomfortable for the patient to maintain this position for a prolonged period and that images may be degraded by artifacts from dental fillings (Fig. 7). These artifacts can often be circumvented by scanning in the subcoronal plane (60° to 80° to Reid's baseline).[24] This subcoronal plane predictably sections the orbit obliquely, but this minor distortion of the structures does not significantly alter the anatomic relationships.

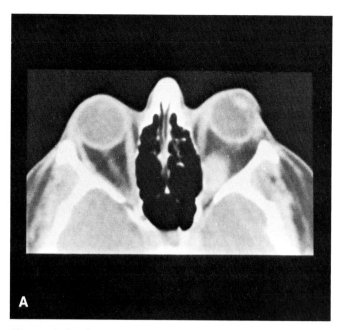

Figure 5.A. Apparent apical mass involving the left orbit.

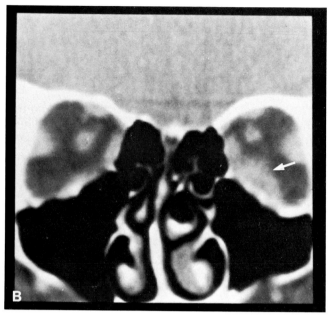

Figure 5.B. Coronal CT reveals enlargement of the inferior rectus muscle of the left orbit (arrow), accounting for the apical mass in A. There is also minimal enlargement of the left medial and lateral rectus muscles. Diagnosis was Graves' disease.

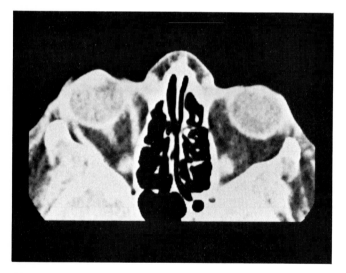

Figure 6. Apparent bilateral apical masses. This is due to oblique sectioning of the normal muscle cone in a plane of section exceeding that of the orbital roof, i.e., approximately +30° to Reid's baseline.

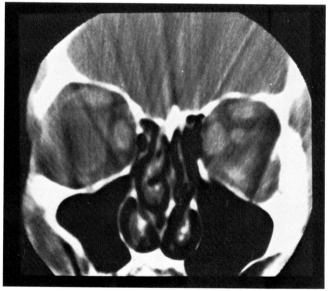

Figure 7. Coronal CT in a patient with extraocular muscle enlargement secondary to Graves' disease. The image is degraded by streak artifacts from dental fillings.

Coronal and sagittal images can also be obtained by direct thin-slice axial scanning with multiplanar reformations.[18,19] Advantages of this approach are that it avoids the head extension, making the procedure more tolerable for the patient. In addition, both coronal and sagittal images can be obtained, and the radiation dose to the lens is slightly less with this method when compared to a study performed with direct axial and direct coronal imaging (see Radiation Dosimetry, below). Disadvantages of this technique are that it takes slightly longer to perform, especially when one takes into account the higher mA and heat-loading demand, requiring longer tube cooling, which is a factor in some CT scanners. In addition, image reformation is somewhat tedious with current software programs, requiring time-consuming computer interaction. A final disadvantage is that there is some loss of anatomic definition with the computer-reformatted displays.

In general, direct axial and direct coronal scanning is the preferred method. The only exception is in trauma cases where a parasagittal view is required to evaluate the orbital floor. In addition, a traumatized patient may not be able to tolerate the hyperextended head position for direct coronals, necessitating the axial sections with computer reformations.

EXTRAOCULAR MUSCLES

There is excellent symmetry between the extraocular muscles in both orbits, and evaluation of their size can be readily performed by comparison. In some disorders of the extraocular muscles, bilateral enlargement commonly occurs, and again, especially with coronal views, this is usually obvious. An apparent subtle enlargement, however, can be more difficult to assess. Measurements are not helpful in view of the normal fusiform configuration of any particular muscle. Slight head rotation may result in a spurious unilateral enlargement. Lateral gaze changes, deliberate or secondary to extraocular nerve palsies or strabismus, result in a contracted muscle on one side, with a relaxed, thinner corresponding muscle in the contralateral orbit (Figs. 8 and 9).

RADIATION DOSIMETRY

The newer generation of CT scanners has not only provided improved image quality, but accomplished this with a lower radiation dose, especially when compared to conventional tomography and early-generation CT scanners utilizing high-resolution techniques. Single-section exposure levels with conventional tomography compare well with those of CT. However, a series of conventional tomographic sections reflects the fact that the radiation passes through all the anatomic layers of the head, irrespective of which layer is in focus. Exposure increases almost arithmetically with the number of contiguous sections obtained.

Computed tomography has a clear advantage over conventional tomography in any series of scans, since the radiation dosage is essentially noncumulative. With the narrow collimation provided in the newer scanners, scatter is minimal, and the dose does not increase by more than a factor of two, regardless of the number of contiguous sections imaged.[25] Further restriction of the total exposure is accomplished with the application of localizer digital radiographs, which themselves only

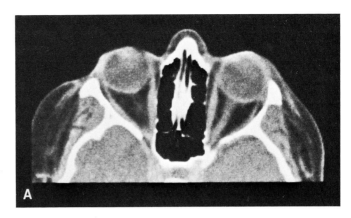

Figure 8. Series of scans demonstrating changes in extraocular muscles secondary to gaze shifts in the same patient.
Figure 8.A. In the primary position of gaze, the extraocular muscles are symmetrical.

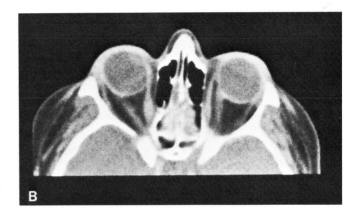

Figure 8.B. Extreme left lateral gaze. This is verified by the position of the optic nerves in the right hand quadrants. The right medial rectus muscle is contracted and thickened. The left medial rectus is relaxed and stretched.

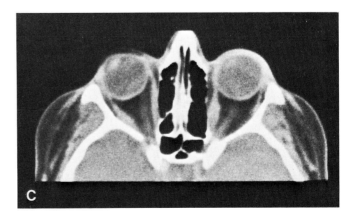

Figure 8.C. Extreme right lateral gaze. The left medial rectus muscle is now contracted, and the right medial rectus relaxed. The right lateral rectus muscle contracted (compared with B).

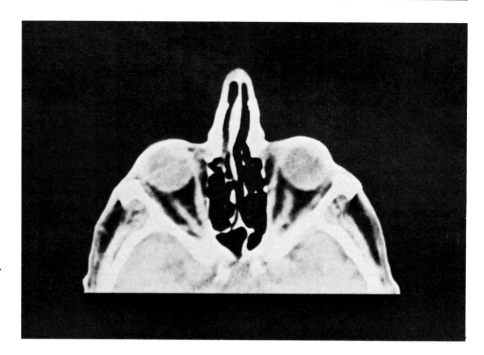

Figure 9. Convergent strabismus on the right, with medial deviation of the right eye, resulting in asymmetry of the medical rectus muscles. Similar medial deviation is found in a sixth nerve or a partial (distal) third nerve palsy.

add approximately 50 to 75 mrad per radiograph to the study.[25]

The following data are pertinent to this discussion. A set of conventional 4-mm complex-motion tomograms to the facial area requiring up to 15 cuts in each of two planes delivers a dose of approximately 30 rad to the facial region (40 kVp, 25 mA, 6 sec). This is contrasted to a series of 5-mm CT sections with 3-mm spacing providing a 2-mm overlap (a technique that can double the speed of the study while allowing adequate resolution for image reformation): a total radiation dose to any section of the patient's face is less than 9 rad.[19]

The critical organ is the ocular lens. In another study,[18] a series of twenty-five 1.5-mm contiguous axial CT scans through the orbit gave a lens dose of 3.6 rad (500 to 600 mA, 576 views, 9.6-sec scans). In this same study, a series of approximately 15 direct axial and direct subcoronal 5-mm scans gave a total lens dose of 5.3 rad (400 mA, 576 views, 9.6-sec scans).

The early generation scanners do not necessarily perform as efficiently. In a study using a rotate-traverse dedicated head scanner in its high-accuracy (slow-speed) mode with overlapping pre- and postcontrast scans, it was found that a potential dose of 40 rad could be delivered to the lens.[26] In view of the availability of high-resolution images with the lower-dose late-generation scanners, utilization of such techniques with older scanners cannot be justified.

REFERENCES

1. Goalwin HA: The precise roentgenography and measurement of the optic canal. AJR 13:480–484, 1925
2. Pfeiffer RL: A new technique for roentgenography of the optic canals. AJR 29:410–415, 1933
3. Hammerschlag SB, O'Reilly GV, Naheedy MH: Computed tomography of the optic canals. AJNR 2:593–594, 1981
4. Carter BL, Morehead J, Wolpert SM, et al: Cross-Sectional Anatomy: Computed Tomography and Ultrasound Correlation. New York, Appelton, 1977, Sect 7
5. Salvolini U, Cabanis EA, Rodallec A, et al: Computed tomography of the optic nerve: Part I. Normal results. J Comput Assist Tomogr 2:141–149, 1978
6. Unsöld R, DeGroot J, Newton TH: Images of the optic nerve: anatomic-CT correlation. AJR 135:767–773, 1980
7. Unsöld R, Newton TH, Hoyt WF: CT examination technique of the optic nerve. J Comput Assist Tomogr 4:560–563, 1980
8. Goalwin HA: One thousand optic canals: a clinical, anatomic and roentgenologic study. JAMA 89:1745–1748, 1927
9. Daniels DL, Haughton VM, Williams AL, Gager WE, Berns TF: Computed tomography of the optic chiasm. Radiology 137:123–127, 1980
10. Haughton VM, Rosenbaum AE, Williams AL, Drayer B: Recognizing the empty sella by CT: the infundibular sign. AJR 136:293–295, 1981
11. Hammerschlag SB, Hughes S, O'Reilly GV, Naheedy MH, Rumbaugh C: Blow-out fractures of the orbit: a comparison of computed tomography and conventional radiography with anatomical correlation. Radiology 143:487–492, 1982
12. Takahashi M, Tamakawa Y: Coronal computed tomography in orbital disease. J Comput Assist Tomogr 1:505–509, 1977
13. Leonardi M, Barbina V, Fabris G, Penco T: Sagittal computed tomography of the orbit. J Comput Assist Tomogr 1:511–512, 1977
14. Wing SD, Hunsaker JN, Anderson RE, Van Dyk HJL, Osborn AG: Direct sagittal computed tomography in

Graves' ophthalmopathy. J Comput Assist Tomogr 3:820–824, 1979

15. Tadmor R, New PFJ: Computed tomography of the orbit with special emphasis on coronal sections. Parts I, II. J Comput Assist Tomogr 2:24–44, 1978

16. Frisén L, Kjällman L, Svendsen P: Computed frontal tomography (CFT) of the orbit using the EMI CT 1010 head scanner. Neuroradiology 15:263–265, 1978

17. Haverling M, Johanson H: Computed sagittal tomography of the orbit. AJR 131:346–347, 1978

18. Forbes GS, Earnest F, Waller RR: Computed tomography of orbital tumors, including late-generation scanning techniques. Radiology 142:387–394, 1982

19. Brant-Zawadzki MN, Minagi H, Federle MP, Rowe LD: High resolution CT with image reformation in maxillofacial pathology. AJNR 3:31–37, 1982

20. Unsöld R, Norman D, Berninger W: Multiplanar evaluation of the optic canal from axial transverse CT sections. J Comput Assist Tomogr 4:418–419, 1980

21. Brismar J, Davis KR, Dallow RC, Brismar G: Unilateral endocrine exophthalmos. Diagnostic problems in association with computed tomography. Neuroradiology 12:21–24, 1976

22. Harris GJ, Syvertsen A: Multiple projection computed tomography in orbital disorders. Ann Ophthalmol 13:183–188, 1981

23. Hammerschlag SB, Wolpert SM, Carter BL: Computed coronal tomography. Radiology 120:219–220, 1976

24. Hesselink JR, New PFJ, Davis KR, et al: Computed tomography of the paranasal sinuses and face: Part I. Normal anatomy. J Comput Assist Tomogr 2:559–567, 1978

25. Maue-Dickson W, Trefler M, Dickson DR: Comparison of dosimetry and image quality in computed and conventional tomography. Radiology 131:509–514, 1979

26. Rice JF, Banks TE: Normal and high accuracy computed tomography of the brain: dose and imaging considerations. J Comput Assist Tomogr 3:497–502, 1979

CHAPTER THREE

The Optic Nerve and Chiasm
Neurofibromatosis

OPTIC NERVE GLIOMAS (Cases 1–13)

Incidence

Optic nerve gliomas are rather uncommon neoplasms, with a general incidence in several large series of 1/175,000 patients presenting with eye complaints.[1-4] Tumor referral centers have a higher incidence, with optic nerve gliomas constituting approximately 3 percent of all intracranial tumors and 4 percent of gliomas.[5-8] Optic nerve gliomas represent 3 percent of orbital tumors.[9] Of the primary optic nerve tumors, optic nerve gliomas outnumber meningiomas three or four to one.[10,11] The sex incidence of optic nerve gliomas is essentially equal.

It has been suggested that optic nerve gliomas are congenital in origin,[2,11,12] although the peak incidence of presentation is from two to six years of age (in the verbal preschool child).[13] Seventy-five percent of cases manifest in the first decade, and 90 percent in the first two decades of life. Rarely, they may occur in middle-aged or older individuals.

Pathologic Features

It will be recalled that the optic nerve is not comparable to other peripheral nerves, but resembles more the pathways of the brain. It differs, however, from the latter by being divided into bundles by extensions of the pial sheath. The fibers themselves are separated by glial tissue that is similar in structure to the glia of the brain. Optic nerve gliomas are therefore essentially brain tumors and almost always are composed of pilocytic (elongated) forms of mature astrocytes[14] consistent with the grade 1 group of astrocytomas. The benign

character and nonprogressive course over a period of years in many cases have led some authors to emphasize the similarities of this lesion to nonneoplastic hamartomas.[12] Optic nerve gliomas expand without invading surrounding tissue.[15] Growth is accounted for by collateral hyperplasia of adjacent glia and connective tissue[2] and production of intra- and extracellular mucosubstance[16] producing microcystic spaces. The absence of mitoses is evidence that these tumors do not enlarge by cell division or invasion.[2] Grossly, they appear as smooth or nodular, fusiform or sausage-shaped intradural enlargement of the optic nerve, which may extend through the optic canal in a dumbbell fashion. They may encroach on the floor of the third ventricle and extend upwards to obstruct the foramen of Monro, producing hydrocephalus. The hypothalamus may be involved and pituitary function may be disturbed. They may extend posteriorly to involve the optic tracts and may even reach the lateral geniculate body.

Optic nerve gliomas have no predilection for any particular site along the optic pathways. At the time of presentation the tumor often appears to have involved an extended region of the optic system. In one recent series of 22 gliomas of the anterior optic pathways evaluated by multiple radiographic techniques including CT, the chiasm was involved in 95 percent cases.[17] Approximately two-thirds of the cases in this series had involvement of the intraorbital optic nerves as well (either unilateral or bilateral). Further evidence for this tendency of transcanalicular extension of optic nerve gliomas was demonstrated in another series[13] by the frequency of optic canal enlargement, which was present in 83 percent of children with optic nerve glioma of one nerve and in 67 percent of those with gliomas involving the chiasm.

Thus, the tumor may occur in any location along the optic pathway, with involvement of the chiasm together with one or both nerves much more common than one nerve alone.

Clinical Manifestations

The most common initial symptom is decreased visual acuity.[13] Intraorbital gliomas manifest relatively early with exophthalmos, which is usually mild. Other presenting symptoms may be nystagmus or strabismus. Chiasmal gliomas may disturb hypothalamic or pituitary function and produce symptoms of increased intracranial pressure. Optic atrophy, papilledema, and variable nonspecific visual field defects may be present. The typical presentation is visual impairment in a verbal preschool child with optic atrophy. Conventional x-ray studies may show concentric enlargement of the involved optic canal with preservation of a well-corticated margin. The sella may be J-shaped due to an eroded chiasmatic sulcus, and the anterior clinoid processes may be deformed.[16]

OPTIC NERVE GLIOMA AND NEUROFIBROMATOSIS (Cases 6–17)

A definite relationship between optic nerve glioma and von Recklinghausen's neurofibromatosis has been established.[18] As opposed to the peripheral form of neurofibromatosis (characterized by subcutaneous nerve sheath tumors with multiple cutaneous café-au-lait spots), optic nerve gliomas are found in the central form of this disorder (characterized by multiple intracranial and intraspinal tumors that arise from the central nervous system parenchyma, its coverings, and the cranial and spinal roots). Although some overlap exists between these forms, patients with the central form usually exhibit few or none of its peripheral stigmata.[14]

The incidence of neurofibromatosis varies considerably among reports of optic nerve gliomas, ranging between 12.3 to 50 percent.[10,13,15,18,19] The large discrepancy in the range of this association is probably accounted for by an underestimation of the frequency of the association of neurofibromatosis and optic nerve glioma at the lower end of the spectrum, due to the usual development of café-au-lait spots at puberty or later, whereas the highest incidence of glioma is in the first decade.[20]

There is no relationship between optic nerve glioma and neurofibromatosis in terms of the anatomic site of the glioma, and the presence of neurofibromatosis does not affect the course or ultimate prognosis of the tumor.[16] The presence of primary optic atrophy in any patient with neurofibromatosis must be highly suspect for having an optic nerve or chiasm glioma.[16,21]

Although optic nerve glioma, neurofibroma, and optic nerve sheath meningioma are all found in patients with neurofibromatosis, coexistence of these tumors is unusual. Enlargement of the optic canal in patients with neurofibromatosis is often secondary to an underlying optic nerve glioma. It may, however, also be secondary to extension of an orbital neurofibroma or, more rarely, to an optic nerve sheath meningioma. Dysplastic bone changes resulting in enlargement of the optic canal without the presence of tumor have also been reported.[15,17]

The orbit may be enlarged as part of the bone dysplasia of neurofibromatosis. An enlarged orbit may also result from an expanding neurofibroma or a large globe secondary to glaucoma. Defects of the sphenoid bone with partial or complete absence of the greater or lesser wings and forward displacement of the middle cranial fossa may also occur as part of the bony dysplasia of neurofibromatosis.[22] Plexiform neurofibromas may involve the eyelids and cause considerable soft-tissue deformity.[18] All of these changes may be detected by CT.

MALIGNANT OPTIC GLIOMA OF ADULTHOOD (Case 18)

Optic gliomas of adulthood differ considerably from optic gliomas of childhood. Malignant astrocytomas of the anterior visual pathways are rare, aggressively invasive, appearing in middle-aged adults, usually males. Within months the patient is totally blind, and death usually occurs in less than a year.[23] The histopathology is that of a glioblastoma multiforme.

CT Manifestations

Any patient with visual loss and a clinical suspicion of an optic system tumor should have the intraorbital optic nerve, optic canal, and the optic chiasm imaged. The method for visualizing the entire anterior pathway has been outlined under the section of technique. It should be emphasized again that the chiasm is optimally scanned in a plane different from that of the intraorbital optic nerve and optic canal. Therefore, a change in gantry tilt or alteration of the head position is necessary to demonstrate all the desired structures.

Intraorbital optic nerve gliomas appear as either a fusiform or sausage-shaped enlargement of the optic nerve. The margins are smooth, and the neoplasm has a sharp interphase with the surrounding orbital fat. Optic nerve gliomas are isodense and have variable enhancement with contrast, often marked. The use of contrast has not been particularly helpful in differentiating optic nerve gliomas from optic nerve sheath meningiomas. Occasionally, optic nerve gliomas may be large and occupy much of the intraconal space. In such cases it becomes difficult to clearly differentiate an optic nerve tumor mass from other intraconal lesions such as a neurilemmoma or a cavernous hemangioma. A large fusiform optic nerve glioma may simulate a cavernous hemangioma. In this instance, contrast enhancement may be helpful, since an enhancing hemangioma can be separated from a normal but displaced optic nerve.

Using a moderately wide window (400 to 500 H units), the diameter of the normal optic nerve in the axial horizontal plane should not exceed 6 mm. Caution should be exercised when measuring in a coronal scan, as a subcoronal plane would tend to exaggerate the cross section due to the obliquity of the angle relative to the axis of the nerve.

A thickened optic nerve is not specific for an optic nerve tumor. Similar appearance is seen in intracranial hypertension with resulting papilledema, optic neuritis, acute central retinal vein occlusion, lymphomatous and leukemic infiltration of the optic nerves, hemangioblastoma, sarcoidosis, advanced Grave's disease, and optic nerve sheath hemorrhage.[24–29]

The optic chiasm and intracranial optic nerves are optimally scanned in a plane parallel or perpendicular to Reid's baseline, with 1.5- or 5-mm sections. A vertical diameter greater than 0.6 cm suggests a chiasmal tumor.[30] Transverse and anteroposterior diameters are less reliable for detecting subtle enlargement. Chiasmal gliomas display variable enhancement. There is usually no difficulty with diagnosis in many cases. The suprasellar mass is obvious, maintaining a characteristic H or X shape of an enlarged chiasm and intracranial optic nerves. Occasionally, even with contrast enhancement, the chiasm, intracranial optic nerves and proximal optic tracts cannot be satisfactorily resolved. In these instances, CT metrizamide cisternography is a useful adjunct, providing a clear definition of these structures.

OPTIC NERVE SHEATH MENINGIOMAS

(Cases 19–27; also see Chapter 5, Cases 10–14 for secondary orbital meningiomas)

Although this discussion relates primarily to optic nerve sheath meningiomas, a brief outline of the various forms of meningiomas that involve the orbit is in order.

Meningiomas encountered in the orbit have several different sites of origin[31–39]:

A. Primary intraorbital meningiomas
   1. Arising from the optic nerve sheath
   2. Arising from ectopic arachnoid cells within the orbit, but unattached to the optic nerve or orbital wall
   3. Arising from the periorbita of the orbital walls
   4. Arising from the optic canal

B. Secondary orbital meningiomas
   1. Arising from the sphenoid wing
   2. Arising from the floor of the anterior cranial fossa with extension into the orbital roof
   3. Perisellar-anterior clinoid area invading the cranio-orbital junction

Incidence

Meningiomas comprise approximately 17 percent of all tumors of the central nervous system. Considering only expanding lesions of the orbit producing unilateral exophthalmos, meningiomas account for only about 5 percent of all lesions.[9,40,41] The large majority of these are secondary orbital meningiomas. Primary intraorbital meningiomas are rare, and most of these have attachment to the optic nerve sheath. Sheath meningiomas occur along the intraoribtal portions of the optic nerve approximately three times more frequently than at the canal.[32] Intracanalicular meningiomas can be as small as a grain of wheat, making diagnosis extremely difficult.

In one series of 25 optic nerve sheath meningiomas, there was a female preponderance similar to that found in central nervous system meningiomas.[31] In this series, 80 percent of tumors occurred in women. The population included both children and the elderly, with a median age of presentation of 38 years. There were two peaks of presentation, one in the 40- to 50-year-old age group, and a second peak in younger individuals. Forty percent occur under age 20, and 24 percent under age 10 years. This earlier presentation of orbital meningiomas compared to intracranial meningiomas is a highly significant clinical feature. Furthermore, primary intraorbital meningiomas in children are more aggressive than similar tumors in adults. There is a higher recurrence rate and poorer survival in children. In young females there is a predilection for involvement of the right orbit. There is also an association with neurofibromatosis in younger individuals, although the central neurofibromatosis may become apparent only after the orbital meningioma has been discovered.

Pathologic Features

An optic nerve sheath meningioma is only partially encapsulated and may extend from its initial subdural site though the dura to involve the extraocular muscles. If it extends under the dura, infiltration along the optic nerve towards the globe or through the optic canal towards the brain may occur. Primary orbital meningiomas are highly invasive but not cytologically malignant. They compress the optic nerve and may invade the sclera. Histologically, they are classified into meningothelial (syncytial) meningiomas comprised of sheets of cells, with oval to vesicular nuclei and distinct cellular outlines, and transitional (mixed) meningiomas, which contain, in addition, spindle cells that are compressed tumor cells at the outskirts of the meningothelial whorls.[31] Psammoma bodies containing calcified concretions are found within the meningiomas but are not a prominent feature.

Clinical Manifestations

The most frequent presenting symptoms are loss of vision with progressive proptosis. Papilledema, chemosis, lid edema, and limitation of ocular motion also occur.[31] Opticociliary venous shunts indicate an optic nerve tumor. Any middle-age woman who develops vision loss and slowly progressive proptosis should be suspect for a meningioma. Also suspect are children with diagnosed or undetected neurofibromatosis who develop proptosis and vision loss. They are at risk to develop either an optic nerve glioma or a meningioma. Cases of atypical optic neuritis that progresses slowly over months or years should be suspect for the diagnosis of intracanalicular meningioma.

Conventional x-ray studies may demonstrate the calcifications within the sheath meningioma. Typically, these appear as a fine cloud-like, stippled conglomeration, parallel lines, or curvilinear whorls of calcification with a central lucency representing the entrapped optic nerve. Foraminal meningiomas may induce hyperostotic bone changes at the orbital apex.[42] Intracanalicular meningiomas may expand the optic canal and produce contour changes with variable cortical thickening. Because of its higher spatial resolution compared to CT, complex-motion tomography is necessary to determine these subtle changes around the optic canal.[43]

CT Manifestations

Optic nerve sheath meningiomas usually manifest as a tubular enlargement of a portion or all of the optic nerve. This contrasts with optic nerve gliomas, which generally result in a fusiform expansion of the optic nerve. This rule, however, is by no means absolute. Both lesions can mimic the other in their general configuration. Meningiomas tend to be slightly hyperdense, whereas gliomas are usually isodense.[44] Meningiomas tend to enhance with contrast more consistently than gliomas. Contrast enhancement in a sheath meningioma may result in a "railroad track" appearance, with the denser tumor surrounding the more lucent central optic nerve. This feature is particularly well seen on coronal views, where the central lucency is more easily identified. Calcification within the lesion strongly favors a meningioma, although occasionally small amounts of calcium may be present in a optic nerve glioma. The meningiomatous calcium may similarly surround a central lucent optic nerve on the coronal views. Both lesions expand the optic canal. However, the presence of hyperostosis around the optic canal is virtually pathognomonic for meningioma. In any one particular case of optic nerve tumor, it may be impossible to differentiate an optic nerve glioma from a sheath meningioma. However, the above-mentioned

CT findings are helpful in making a more definitive diagnosis in many cases.

Other Optic Nerve Disorders (Cases 28–32)

Optic atrophy, optic neuritis, and papilledema are illustrated in Cases 28–32. See also Chapter 7, Cases 21, 25, and 36.

REFERENCES

1. Collins F, Marshall D: Two cases of primary neoplasm of the optic nerves. Trans Ophthal Soc UK 20:156–164, 1900
2. Verhoeff FH: Primary intraneural tumors of the optic nerve. Arch Ophthalmol 51:120–140, 239–254, 1922
3. Boles WM, Naugle TC, Sanson CLM: Glioma of the optic nerve. Report of a case arising from the optic disc. Arch Ophthalmol 59:229–231, 1958
4. Arkhangelski UN: Neoplasm of the optic nerve. Ophthalmologica 151:260–271, 1966
5. Martin P, Cushing H: Primary gliomas of the chiasm and optic nerves in their intracranial portions. Arch Ophthalmol 52:209–241, 1923
6. Taveras JM, Mount LA, Wood EH: The value of radiation therapy in the management of glioma of the optic nerves and chiasm. Radiology 66:518–528, 1956
7. Fowler FD, Matson DD: Gliomas of the optic pathways in childhood. J Neurosurg 14:515–528, 1957
8. Matson DD: Neurosurgery of infancy and childhood, Springfield, Ill., Charles C Thomas, 1969
9. Reese AB: Tumors of the Eye, 2nd ed. New York, Harper & Row, Hoeber Medical, 1963
10. Davis FA: Primary tumors of the optic nerve (a phenomenon of Recklinghausen's disease): a clinical and pathological study with a report of five cases and a review of the literature. Arch Ophthalmol 23:735–821, 957–1022, 1940
11. Hudson AC: Primary tumors of the optic nerve. Royal London Ophthalmol Hosp Rep 18:317–439, 1912
12. Hoyt WF, Baghdassarian SA: Optic glioma of childhood. Natural history and rationale for conservative management. Br J Ophthalmol 53:793–798, 1969
13. Chutorian AM, Schwartz JF, Evans RA; Carter S: Optic gliomas in children. Neurology 14:83–95, 1964
14. Rubinstein LJ: Tumors of the central nervous system, 2nd ser, fasicle 6. Washington, DC, Armed Forces Institute of Pathology, 1972
15. Christensen E, Anderson SR: Primary tumours of the optic nerve and chiasm. Acta Psychiatr Neurol Scand 27:5–16, 1952
16. Anderson DR, Spencer WH: Ultrastructure and histochemical observations of optic nerve gliomas. Arch Ophthalmol 83:324–335, 1970
17. Savoiardo M, Harwood-Nash DC, Tadmor R, Scotti G, Musgrave MA: Gliomas of the intracranial anterior optic pathways in children. The role of computed tomography, angiography, pneumoencephalography and radionuclide brain scanning. Radiology 138:601–610, 1981
18. Marshall D: Glioma of the optic nerve (as a manifestation of von Recklinghausen's disease) Am J Ophthalmol 37:15–36, 1954

19. Burki E: Uber den primaren Sehnerventumor und seine Beziehungen zur Recklinghausenschen Neurofibromatose. Bibl Ophthalmol (Basel) 30, 1944

20. Eggers H, Jakobiec FA, Jones IS: Tumors of the optic nerve. Doc Ophthalmol 41(1):43–128, 1976

21. Dresner F, Montgomery DAD: Primary optic atrophy in von Recklinghausen's disease. Q J Med 18:93–103, 1949

22. Burrows EH: Bone changes in orbital neurofibromatosis. Br J Radiol 36:549–561, 1963

23. Hoyt WF, Meshel LG, Lessell S, Schatz NJ: Malignant optic glioma of adulthood. Brain 96: 121–132, 1973

24. Tourje EJ, Gola LHA: Leukemic infiltration of the optic nerves: demonstration by computed tomography. Comput Tomogr 1: 225–228, 1977

25. Statton R, Blodi FC; Hanigan J: Sarcoidosis of the optic nerve. Arch Ophthalmol 71:834–836, 1964

26. Cananis EA, Salvolini U, Rodallec A. et al: Computed tomography of the optic nerve: Part II. Size and shape modifications in papilledema. J Comput Assist Tomogr 2:150–155, 1978

27. Lauten GJ, Eatherly JB, Ramirez A: Hemangioblastoma of the optic nerve: Radiographic and pathologic features. AJNR 2:96–99, 1981

28. Trokel SL, Hilal SK. Recognition and differential diagnosis of enlarged extraocular muscles in computed tomography. Am J Ophthalmol 87:503–512, 1979

29. Muller PJ, Deck JHN. Intraocular and optic nerve sheath hemorrhage in cases of sudden intracranial hypertension. J Neurosurg 41:160–166, 1974

30. Daniels DL, Haughton VM, Williams AL, Gager WE, Berns TF: Computed tomography of the optic chiasm. Radiology 137:123–127, 1980

31. Karp LA, Zimmerman LE, Borit A, Spencer W: Primary intraorbital meningiomas. Arch Ophthalmol 91:24–28, 1974

32. Craig WM, Gogela LJ: Intraorbital meningiomas. A clinicopathologic study. Am J Ophthalmol 32:1663–1680, 1949

33. Tan KK, Lin SM: Primary extradural intraorbital meningioma in a Chinese girl. Br J Ophthalmol 49:377–380, 1965

34. Macmichael IM, Cullen JF: Primary intraorbital meningioma. Br J Ophthalmol 53:169–173, 1969

35. Mandelcorn MS, Shea M: Primary orbital perioptic meningioma. Can J Ophthalmol 6:293–297, 1971

36. D'Alena P: Primary orbital meningioma. Arch Ophthalmol 71:832–833, 1964

37. Sanders MD, Falconer MA: Optic nerve compression by an intracanalicular meningioma. Br J Ophthalmol 48:13–18, 1964

38. Gordon E: Orbital extension of meningioma. Can J Ophthalmol 5:381–385, 1970

39. Sterns WE: Meningiomas of the cranio-orbital junction. J Neurosurg 38:428–437, 1973

40. Reese AB: Expanding lesions of the orbit. Trans Ophthalmol Soc UK 91:85–104, 1971

41. Reese AB: Incidence and management of unilateral proptosis. In Boniuk M (ed): Ocular and Adrenal Tumors. St. Louis, CV Mosby, 1964, pp 389–394

42. Lloyd GAS: The radiology of primary orbital meningioma. Br J Radiol 44:405–411, 1971

43. Strother CM, Hoyt WF, Appen RE, Newton TH. Meningiomatous changes in the optic canal. A polytomographic study. Radiology 135:109–114, 1980

44. Forbes GS, Sheedy PF, Waller RR: Orbital tumors evaluated by computed tomography. Radiology 136:101–111, 1980

CASE 1. Optic Nerve Glioma

A 32-year-old male with increasing blurred vision and inferior field defect on the right progressive over 2 years, accompanied by a right temporal headache and mild intermittent irritation of the right eye. Visual acuity: 20/70 OD, 20/20 OS. The visual field in the right eye showed a dense inferior altitudinal defect with extension in the upper temporal quadrant. Visual field on the left was normal. Color perception OD was decreased. Exophthalmometer readings: 23.5 OD and 19.0 OS at base 102. The right eye was proptosed straight forward, with increased resistance on retropulsion. Ocular motility was full. There was an afferent pupillary defect and moderately advanced optic atrophy. Left eye and orbit were normal.

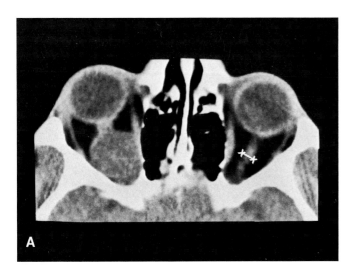

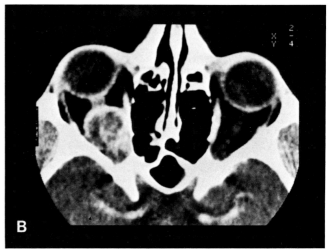

Figure A. There is a fusiform expansion of the right optic nerve occupying the posterior orbit. The optic nerve is thickened up to the globe. Mild proptosis is present. The left optic nerve is normal (cursor).

Figure B. With contrast, there is inhomogeneous enhancement.

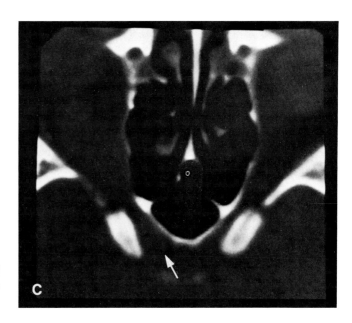

Figure C. CT of the optic canals demonstrates marked expansion of the entire right optic canal (arrow), indicating transcanalicular spread of the tumor.

Follow-up: The patient underwent craniotomy and orbitotomy, which revealed a large tumor extending from the junction of the optic nerve and the globe posteriorly through the optic canal and involving the chiasm and optic tract on the right side, with extension into the hypothalamus. Biopsy revealed glioma. The tumor was amputated 2-mm anterior to the chiasm and at the posterior globe with removal of this segment. The residual intracranial tumor was treated with radiation therapy.

CASE 2. Optic Nerve Glioma

A 17-year-old female with 3-year history of deteriorating vision on the left.

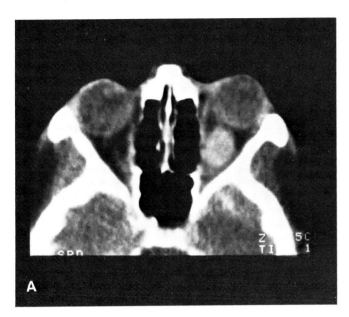

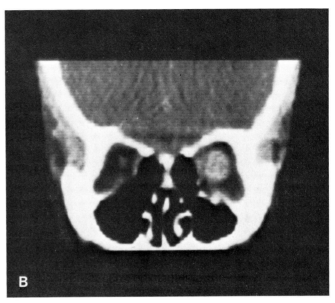

Figure A. CT with contrast demonstrates an enhancing fusiform-shaped left optic nerve.

Figure B. Coronal CT with contrast confirms that the enhancing mass is located centrally, indicating that it represents an enlarged optic nerve.

Follow-up: Orbital exploration via a frontal craniotomy confirmed an optic nerve glioma confined to the orbit, without transcanalicular extension.

CASE 3. Optic Nerve Glioma

A seven-year-old female with two-month history of decreasing vision and prominence of left eye. Visual acuity: 20/25 OD, fingers at one foot OS. Hertel measurements were 11 on right; 17, left. The left eye also demonstrated resistance to retropulsion, an afferent pupillary defect, and a pale elevated blurred disc. The right eye was normal.

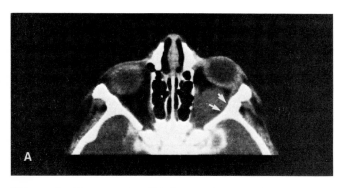

Figure A. Noncontrast CT demonstrates a fusiform expansion of the left optic nerve. Note the scalloped appearance of the orbital surface of the sphenoid wing (arrows) secondary to the expanding mass.

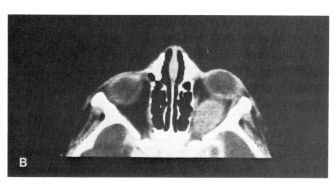

Figure B. Following intravenous contrast administration, the optic nerve glioma enhances approximately 30 H units. Although this delineates the mass better, no significant additional information has been gained.

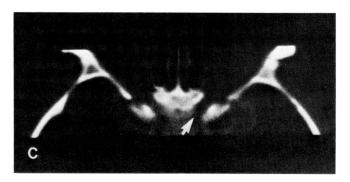

Figure C. CT of the optic canals with bone windows. The left canal (arrow) is significantly larger than the right, indicating transcanalicular extension of the tumor.

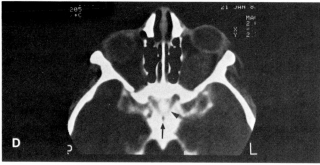

Figure D. CT metrizamide cisternogram. The intracranial optic nerve immediately anterior to the optic chiasm (arrowhead) is normal, as is the chiasm itself. The infundibulum (arrow) is located immediately posterior to the chiasm.

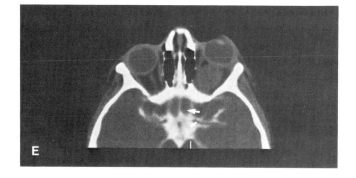

Figure E. CT section slightly craniad to D. The gyrus rectus (large arrow) is seen anterior to the chiasm. The optic tract (small arrow) is seen extending posteriorly from the chiasm.

Diagnosis: Optic nerve glioma with transcanalicular extension, but without involvement of the optic chiasm.

CASE 4. Optic System Glioma

This 15-month-old male was first noted to have nystagmus and decreased visual responsiveness at age 4 months. Examination at 15 months revealed bilateral optic atrophy, poor fixation, nystagmus, and markedly decreased visual acuity. At the time of diagnosis there was no evidence of any cutaneous manifestations of neurofibromatosis.

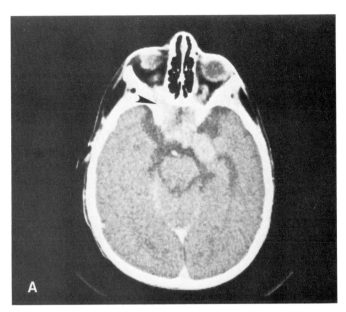

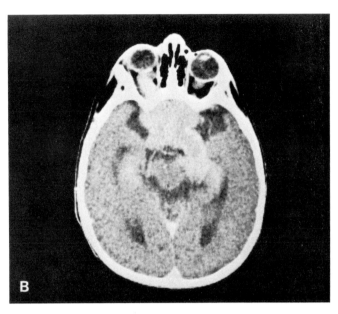

Figure A. CT at the level of the anterior clinoid processes demonstrates an enhancing suprasellar mass eroding into the sphenoid sinus anteriorly and laterally into the intracranial ends of the optic canals, particularly on the right (arrowhead). Masses are identified in both orbital apices.*

Figure B. CT slightly more craniad than in A demonstrates a markedly thickened right optic nerve. The left optic nerve is only partially seen and is also thickened.

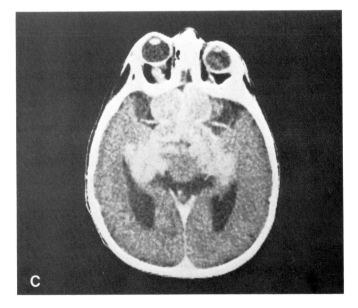

Figure C. CT more craniad than B outlines the entire intracranial extent of the tumor. The optic chiasm and hypothalamic region are markedly enlarged due to tumor involvement, with thickening of both intracranial optic nerves anterior to the chiasm. Posterior to the chiasm, both optic tracts are involved with extension up to the lateral geniculate bodies. Hydrocephalus is present as demonstrated by enlarged atria and temporal horns of the lateral ventricles.

Follow-up: On the basis of the clinical and CT findings, the patient was treated with 4000 rads of radiation therapy.

*Reprinted from Hesselink JR, Weber AL: Pathways of orbital extension of extraorbital neoplasms. J Comput Assist Tomogr 6:596, 1982, with permission.

CASE 5. Optic Chiasm–Hypothalamic Glioma

This 32-year-old male had a 5-year history of dizzy spells. He recently developed a left temporal field defect. Examination: Left temporal hemianopsia. *Vision:* 20/40 OU. Bilateral optic atrophy. Pupils normal.

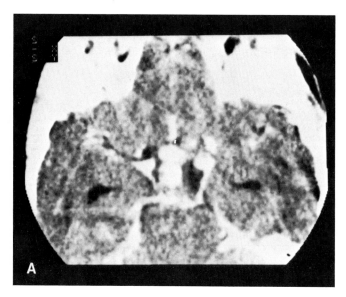

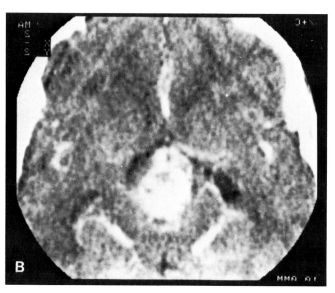

Figure A. Axial CT through the suprasellar cistern demonstrates a bilobed suprasellar enhancing mass, surrounded by the circle of Willis vessels. Laterally the temporal horns are dilated.

Figure B. Section slightly craniad to A. The enhancing mass fills the suprasellar cistern and extends posteriorly into the interpeduncular cistern.

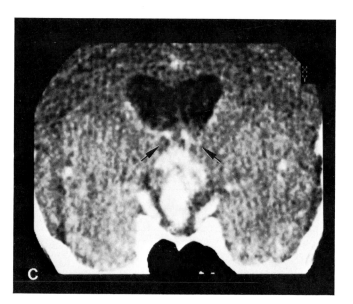

Figure C. Coronal CT shows the vertical extent of the chiasmatic tumor. Inferiorly it projects into the sella; superiorly it has obliterated the anterior third ventrical and abuts on the interventricular foramen (arrows). The lateral ventricals are enlarged due to the obstruction at the foramen of Monro.

Follow-up: Surgery via a right subfrontal craniotomy revealed an optic chiasm–hypothalamic tumor. Histologic examination: juvenile pilocytic glioma.

CASE 6. Neurofibromatosis and Optic Nerve Glioma

A three-year-old male with florid cutaneous neurofibromatosis with muscle incoordination. Minimal right proptosis. Visual acuity normal. Visual fields full to confrontation. Fundi were normal without papilledema or optic atrophy.

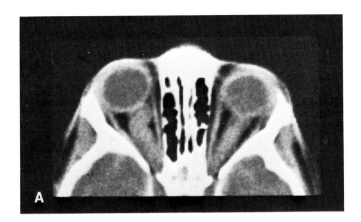

Figure A. CT of the orbits demonstrates marked thickening of both optic nerves, more prominent on the right.

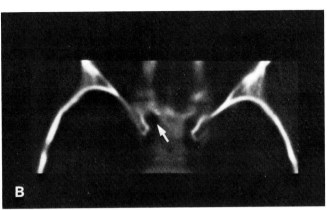

Figure B. CT through optic canals with bone windows demonstrates enlarged optic canals bilaterally, more prominent on the right (arrow).

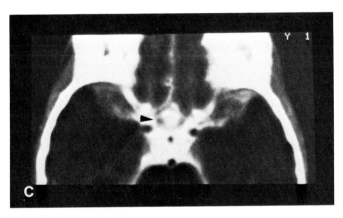

Figure C. CT metrizamide cisternogram through the suprasellar cistern. Both intracranial optic nerves are clearly delineated. The right nerve (arrowhead) is enlarged. The left nerve is borderline enlarged.

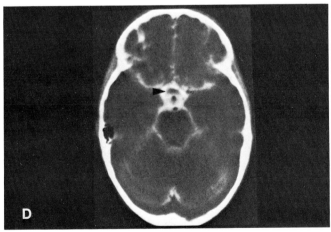

Figure D. CT metrizamide cisternogram, section slightly more craniad than C. The optic chiasm is slightly prominent, with asymmetric enlargement of the right side (arrowhead).

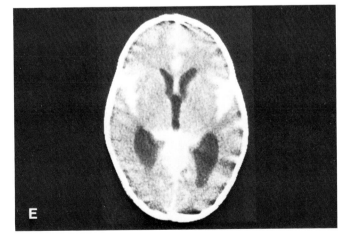

Figure E. CT metrizamide study. The lateral and third ventricles are mildly enlarged. No contrast has entered the ventricular system. A subsequent ventriculogram revealed aqueductal stenosis.

Diagnosis: Neurofibromatosis with optic system glioma (no histologic confirmation). An unusual feature of this case is the preserved vision with profound pathologic changes.

CASE 7. Neurofibromatosis and Optic Nerve Glioma
A two-year-old female with neurofibromatosis and enlarging left optic canal by serial x-ray examinations. There was left-sided proptosis.

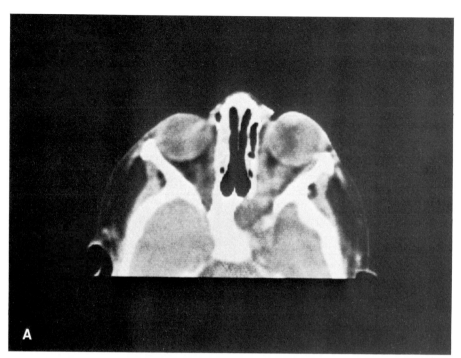

Figure A. CT demonstrates a thick left optic nerve extending into an enlarged optic canal.

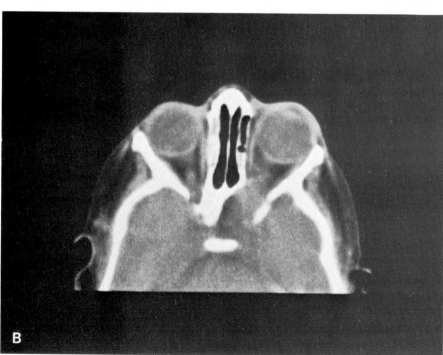

Figure B. CT slightly craniad to A demonstrates a markedly enlarged optic canal with erosion medially into the sphenoid sinus and posterior ethmoid sinus.

Follow-up: Patient was referred for radiation therapy.

CASE 8. Neurofibromatosis and Optic Nerve Glioma

This two-year-old female had decreased vision left eye and progressive proptosis. Fundoscopy revealed optic atrophy on the left.

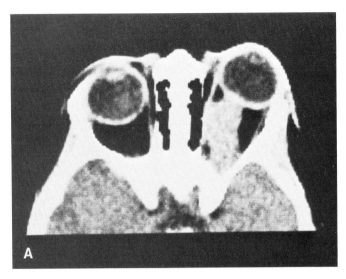

Figure A. Initial CT demonstrates a large hyperdense left optic nerve tumor that appears to have an exophytic component medially. There is considerable proptosis.

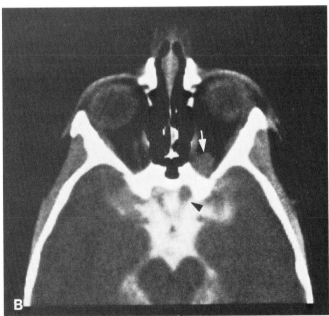

Figure B. Following excision of the intraorbital optic nerve (performed to relieve the proptosis), a subsequent CT metrizamide cisternogram demonstrates residual tumor in the orbital apex (arrow). The left intracranial optic nerve, surrounded by contrast, is considerably thickened (arrowhead), indicating involvement with tumor. However, the optic chiasm and right intracranial nerve are of normal caliber.

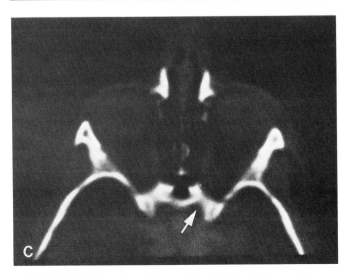

Figure C. CT of the optic canals with bone windows demonstrate enlargement of the left canal (arrow).

CASE 9. Optic Nerve Glioma

An eight-year-old female who presented with visual loss. Visual acuity: 20/20 OD; no light perception on the left. Left optic atrophy was present.

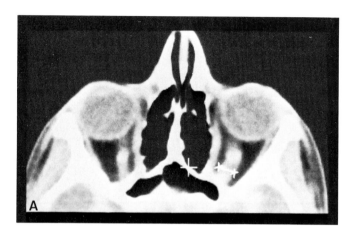

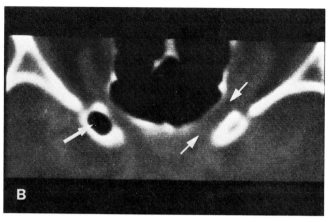

Figure A. CT reveals thickened left optic nerve (cursor), which enhanced approximately 20 H units with contrast administration.

Figure B. CT of the optic canals reveals diffuse enlargement of the left optic canal (small arrows). The black density (large arrow) is an aerated right anterior clinoid process.

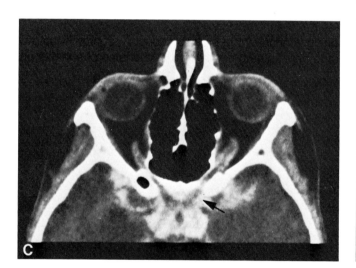

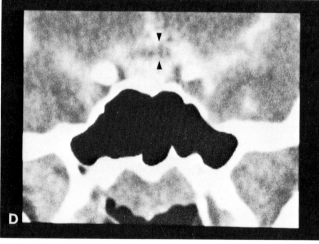

Figure C. CT metrizamide cisternogram outlines the suprasellar structures. The left intracranial optic nerve (arrow) is slightly thickened when compared to the contralateral side. Metrizamide outlines both the intraorbital optic nerves, indicating the CSF communication between the intracranial basal cisterns and the intraorbital perioptic subarachnoid space. In view of the expanded left optic nerve and enlarged optic canal, it is difficult to comprehend how the perioptic subarachnoid space has remained patent.

Figure D. Coronal CT metrizamide cisternogram outlines the optic chiasm, which is slightly thickened on the left side (arrowheads).

Diagnosis: Optic nerve glioma with involvement of the intraorbital and intracranial optic nerve and the optic chiasm (no histologic confirmation).

CASE 10. Neurofibromatosis with Optic Nerve Glioma and Orbit Neurofibroma

A 23-year-old female with neurofibromatosis. At age 6 years she underwent a left orbital exploration via a transcranial approach, which revealed an apparent optic nerve glioma. Postoperatively she received radiation therapy. She now presents with increasing left proptosis. Vision has been poor since age 6, with no recent deterioration. Examination revealed the left eye to be displaced downwards by an upper nasal quadrant mass. Proptosis of 4 mm was present on the left. Extraocular movements were all limited on the left. Fundoscopy revealed a pale left disk with normal vessels.

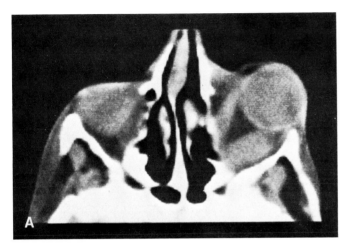

Figure A. Axial CT at the level of the inferior orbit demonstrates proptotic left eye. The left optic nerve is moderately thickened.

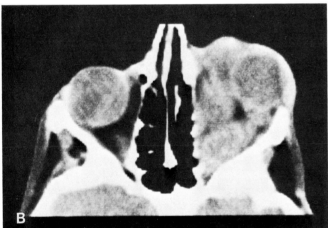

Figure B. CT section craniad to A again demonstrates the thickened left optic nerve, which occupies the orbital apex and extends to the laterally displaced globe. Medial to this is second soft-tissue mass (neurofibroma) that extends from the retrobulbar space to bulge out anteriorly, adjacent to the globe.

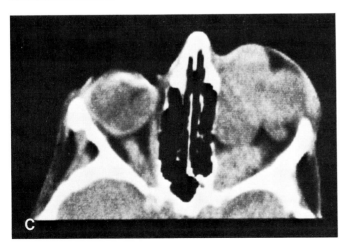

Figure C. CT section craniad to B again defines the medially located neurofibroma. It has well-defined sharp margins. The tortuous optic nerve glioma is posterior and lateral to the neurofibroma. Note that the entire left orbit is enlarged, and the left ethmoid sinus is slightly smaller than the right. These changes are most likely related to the bony dysplasia of neurofibromatosis, although the soft-tissue masses could contribute to the orbital expansion.

CASE 11. Neurofibromatosis, Optic Nerve Glioma, and Congenital Glaucoma

A three-year-old female with neurofibromatosis, exophthalmos, and blind left eye.

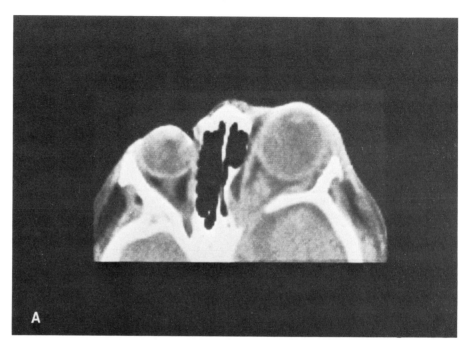

Figure A. The left orbit is much larger than the right. There is a defect in the left sphenoid wing, and the sphenoid wing is located more anteriorly on the left, enlarging the adjacent middle cranial fossa. The left ethmoid sinus is reduced in size. The globe is markedly enlarged due to the glaucoma. The optic nerve appears thickened.

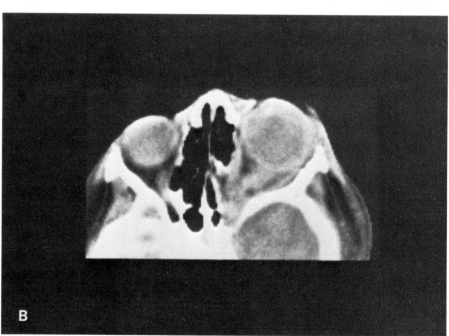

Figure B. This section defines the left optic nerve better. It is enlarged, consistent with an optic nerve glioma (no histologic confirmation).

CASE 12. Neurofibromatosis and Intracranial Optic System Glioma

An eight-year-old male with café-au-lait spots and neurofibromatosis. At age one year, he was noted to have left-side papilledema and enlarged left optic foramen. A pneumoencephalogram performed at that time was negative. Diagnosed as an optic nerve glioma but not treated. At age five years, he developed intermittent headaches. Bilateral optic atrophy was present. CT revealed a suprasellar mass. The patient was not treated at that time. Recently, he presented with precocious puberty.

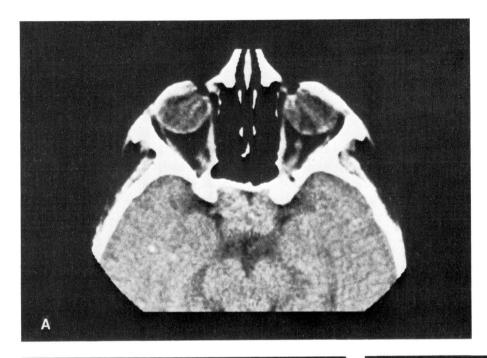

Figure A. CT with contrast through the suprasellar cistern demonstrates a markedly enlarged optic chiasm and involvement of both intracranial optic nerves.

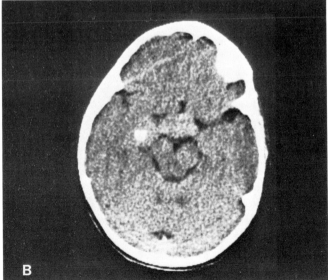

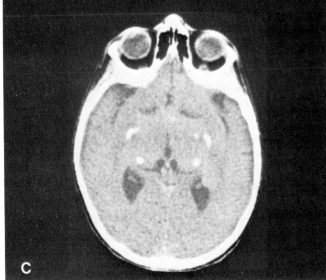

Figure B. CT section slightly more craniad than A shows large suprasellar tumor involving optic chiasm and hypothalamic region. The tumor extends into the right optic tract, as evidenced by increased density and calcium.

Figure C. The full extent of the tumor is demonstrated by calcifications involving both optic tracts extending posteriorly up to the region of the lateral geniculate bodies.

Follow-up: Patient underwent radiation therapy. The signs of precocious puberty decreased shortly after initiating the therapy.

CASE 13. Neurofibromatosis with Optic System Glioma
This nine-year-old female had neurofibromatosis and decreased vision.

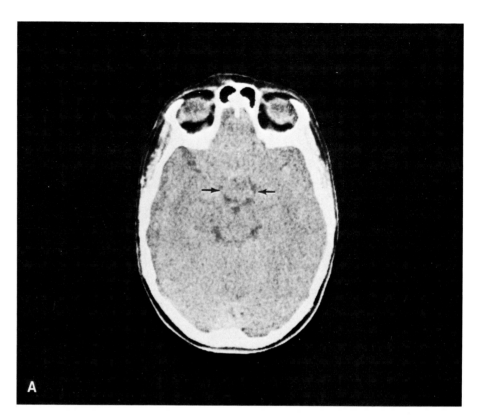

Figure A. The suprasellar cistern is filled with a mass representing an enlarged optic chiasm (arrows), which is isodense with the surrounding brain (this is a noncontrast study).

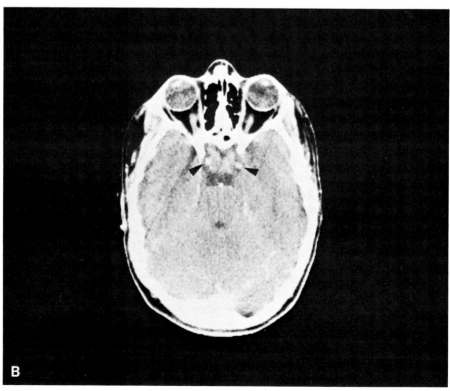

Figure B. Contrast-enhanced study, with sections slightly caudade to A, demonstrates mild enhancement of the chiasmatic tumor. There is involvement of both intracranial optic nerves, as well as the right intraorbital optic nerve. The circular densities on either side of the optic chiasm represent the internal carotid arteries (arrowheads). In view of the clear delineation of the suprasellar tumor in this case, CT metrizamide cisternography would not provide any additional significant information.

CASE 14. Neurofibromatosis with Glaucoma

A two-year-old male with neurofibromatosis (strong family history). Noted to have bulging left eyeball at age 10 months. Vision reported as good. There was no clinical suspicion for an optic nerve glioma. The left cornea and iris were much larger than the right, with unusual pigmentation involving the right iris.

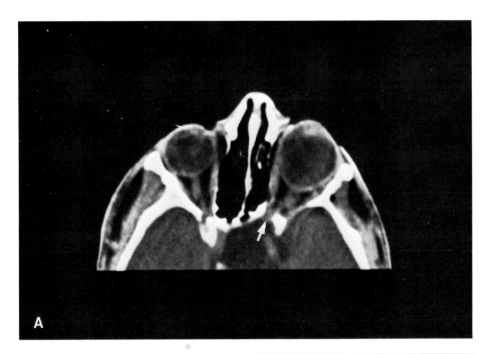

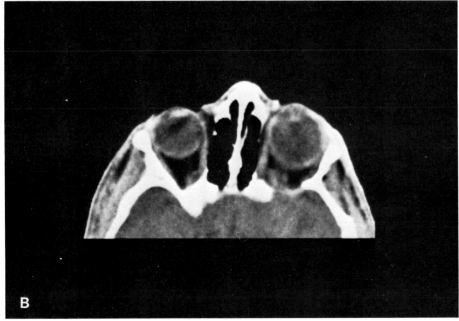

Figures A and B. Two contiguous CT sections demonstrate a large left orbit with a defect involving the greater wing of the sphenoid. The middle lobe of the brain does not herniate into the orbit. The ethmoid sinus is reduced in size on the left. The optic canal is enlarged (arrow), and the region of the left chiasmatic sulcus extends more anteriorly on the left (providing a J-shaped sella on the lateral skull x-ray). The left anterior clinoid process is small. The left optic nerve appears slightly thickened, suggesting optic nerve glioma. No suprasellar mass was identified. The perisellar bony changes, including the enlarged optic canal, are probably part of the bone dysplasia of neurofibromatosis and are unrelated to transcanalicular tumor growth, although this cannot be stated with absolute certainty.

Follow-up: Patient was treated with gonial curettage of the medial angle of the left eye for control of glaucoma.

CASE 15. Neurofibromatosis

A five-year-old female with neurofibromatosis diagnosed in infancy. She has glaucoma involving the right eye, for which she has had three goniotomy procedures, all of which failed to control the increased intraocular pressure. Over the past three years she developed a right upper lid mass with ptosis, as well as progressive proptosis.

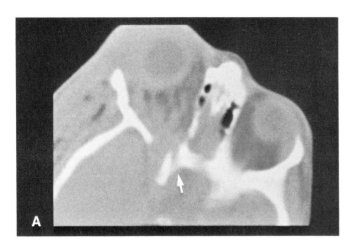
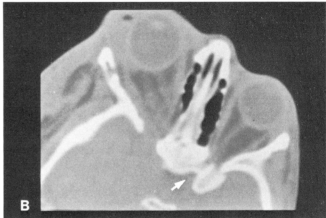

Figures A and B. CT with bone windows demonstrates the skeletal deformities. The right orbit is much larger than the left, with concomitant reduction in the size of the right ethmoid labyrinth. There is a defect involving the greater and lesser wings of the sphenoid bone. The optic canals are identified on sequential sections (arrows). The right optic canal is probably slightly larger than the left in its midcanalicular part. All of these changes described can be accounted for on the basis of the bony dysplasia associated with neurofibromatosis.

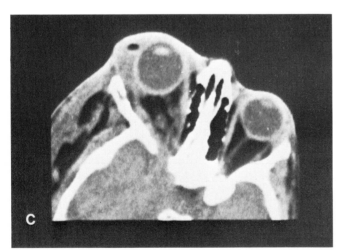
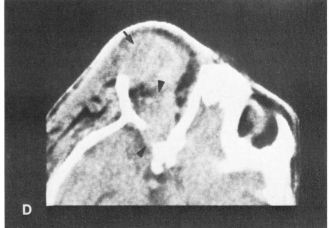

Figure C. The right ocular bulb is larger than the left due to the glaucoma. There is a soft-tissue mass anteriorly and anterolaterally, representing a plexiform neurofibroma of the upper lid. The air bubble anteriorly is under the upper lid. Excessive soft tissue is seen posteriorly. This is better defined in D.

Figure D. This section is more craniad than C. There is a significant retrobulbar soft-tissue mass (arrowheads) that extends through the defect in the sphenoid wing and most likely is a neurofibroma, accounting for the progressive proptosis. The anteriorly located plexiform neurofibroma (arrow) extends over the globe.

Diagnosis: Neurofibromatosis with orbital bony abnormalities, glaucoma, plexiform neurofibroma of the upper lid, and probable retrobulbar neurofibroma (no histologic confirmation).

CASE 16. Neurofibromatosis with Plexiform Neurofibroma of the Upper Lid

This two-year-old female had neurofibromatosis with a soft-tissue mass of the upper lid producing ptosis. Skull x-ray revealed a large right orbit and abnormal sella.

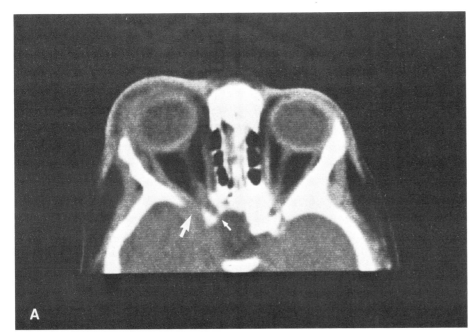

Figure A. The right orbit is enlarged. There is a defect involving the sphenoid wing (large arrow), and the right middle cranial fossa is expanded due to the more anterior location of the sphenoid wing. The right optic canal is prominent (small arrow). Immediately adjacent to it, the sella is expanded, with the bony defect extending into the basisphenoid. All of the bony changes are on the basis of the dysplasia of neurofibromatosis. The optic nerve appears normal.

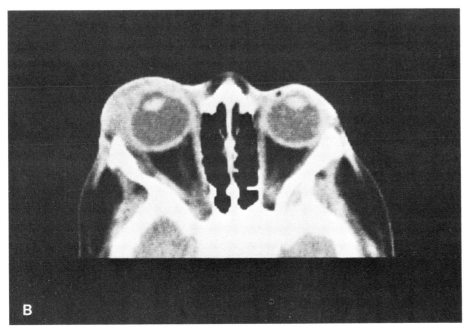

Figure B. The soft-tissue mass anterior to the right globe represents a plexiform neurofibroma of the upper lid.

CASE 17. Neurofibromatosis with Plexiform Neurofibroma
A 49-year-old male with 20-year history of left exophthalmos. A left orbital plexiform neurofibroma was diagnosed at the outset, with several subsequent debulking procedures. Examination revealed left eye to be 13 mm more prominent than the right. Visual acuity was 20/20 OU. Orbital resilience markedly decreased on the left. A firm mass was palpable beneath the left upper lid near the superior temporal rim.

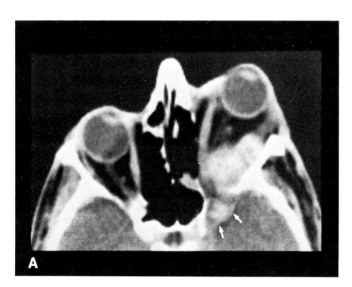

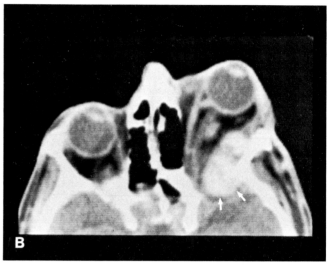

Figure A. There is marked proptosis. The left orbital is considerably enlarged when compared to the right. A defect in the sphenoid wing is evident. A well-defined, enhancing soft-tissue mass (the plexiform neurofibroma) occupies the orbital apex and extends postero-laterally along the sphenoid wing. This mass has extended through the bony defect into the middle cranial fossa (arrows). The medial rectus muscle appears thickened.

Figure B. CT section slightly craniad to A. The enhancing plexiform neurofibroma protrudes through the sphenoid wing defect (arrows), bulging into the middle cranial fossa. The optic nerve is stretched and bowed medially.

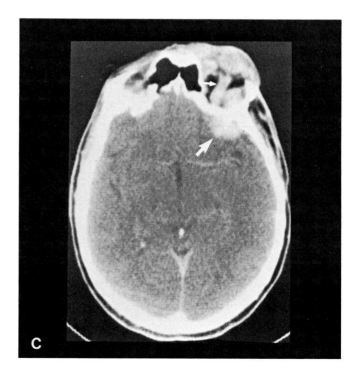

Figure C. CT section through the superior left orbit. The enhancing plexiform neurofibroma bulges into the anterior cranial fossa (large arrow). The superior rectus muscle (small arrow) is prominent.

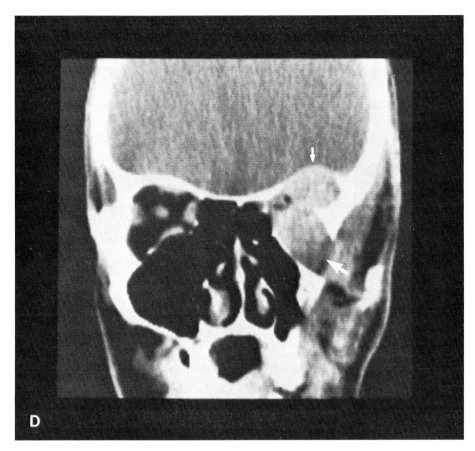

D

Figure D. Coronal section at the level of the posterior orbit. Much of the left orbit is occupied by the soft-tissue mass, with erosion of the roof (small arrow), as well as extension into a widened inferior orbital fissure (large arrow). The left ethmoid and maxillary sinuses are compressed.

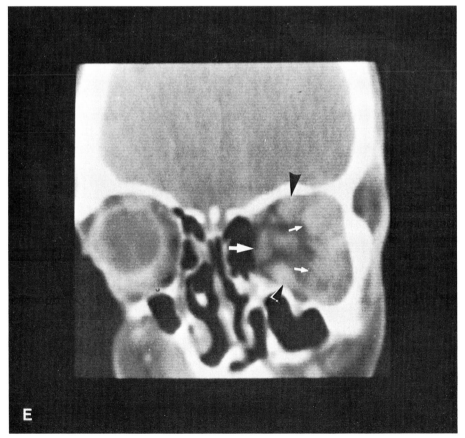

E

Figure E. Coronal section at the level of the anterior orbit. The expanded left orbit is again appreciated. The extraconal soft-tissue mass (small arrows) occupies the superotemporal quadrant. The extraocular muscles are thickened (superior rectus–levator palpebrae superioris complex = large black arrowhead; inferior rectus = small black arrowhead; medial rectus = large arrow). The optic nerve in the center appears thickened, but this central density is a combination of normal optic nerve and an adjacent structure (see B), which is probably a dilated vein.

Diagnosis: Neurofibromatosis with bony dysplasia of orbit and retrobulbar plexiform neurofibroma. The thickened extraocular muscles are probably secondary to the apical mass with compression and congestion of the muscles.

CASE 18. Malignant Optic Nerve Glioma (Glioblastoma Multiforme)
An 80-year-old male with rapid loss of vision in the left eye over a period of five weeks. At 2½ months from the initial onset, he was totally blind in both eyes. At fundoscopy the tumor could be visualized at the left optic disc. Surgical exploration via a frontal craniotomy demonstrated a markedly thickened optic chiasm and intracranial optic nerves, more prominent on the left. Biopsy revealed glioblastoma multiforme.

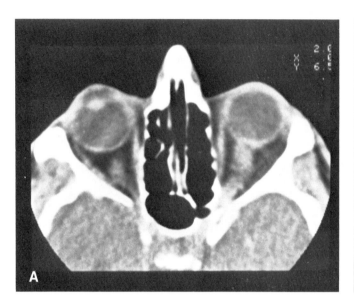

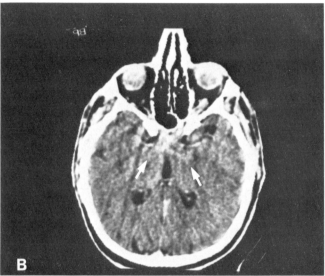

Figure A. Initial CT scan demonstrates a diffusely thickened left optic nerve, extending up to the optic nerve head.

Figure B. Scan several weeks later reveals an enlarged enhancing optic chiasm and intracranial nerves. The thickened left optic nerve also enhances. There is involvement of both optic tracts (arrows), more prominent on the left. A CT scan of the optic canals revealed no enlargement.

Follow-up: The patient underwent radiation treatment: 4000 rad was given to the optic chiasm and optic nerves. Five weeks later he developed an expressive aphasia.

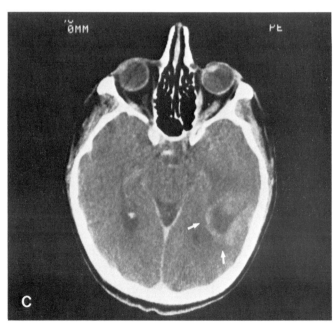

Figure C. Repeat scan with contrast enhancement at follow-up demonstrates that the tumor has spread to the left posterior temporal region (arrows) with surrounding edema.

CASE 19. Optic Nerve Sheath Meningioma

A 69-year-old female with deteriorating vision in the left eye for a year. Visual acuity: Hand movements at three feet OS, 20/20 OD. Inferior altitudinal defect and afferent pupillary defect OS. OD normal. No proptosis. Ocular motility intact. Fundoscopy: Optic atrophy OS without abnormal shunt vessels or retinal striae. OD fundus normal. Examination 18 months later: OS no light perception. Two millimeters of exophthalmos OS with reduced orbital resilience.

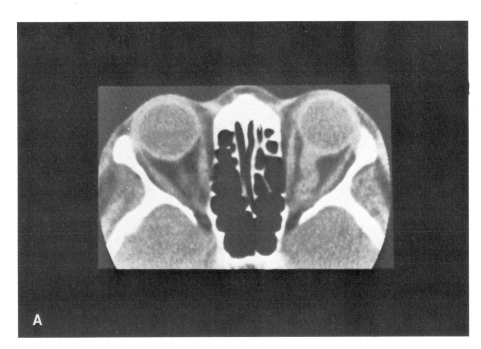

Figure A. There is a tubular expansion of the entire intraorbital optic nerve on the left. The nerve has assumed a tortuous configuration to accommodate its increased bulk.

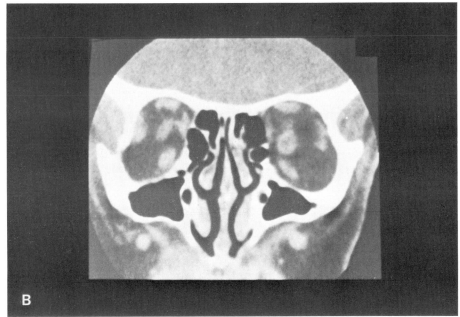

Figure B. Coronal CT demonstrates the enlarged left optic nerve. The periphery of the nerve is dense relative to the central lucency. This finding is good evidence for an optic nerve sheath meningioma surrounding the optic nerve, which is represented by the central lucency.

CASE 20. Optic Nerve Sheath Meningioma
A 65-year-old female with decreased visual acuity and a field defect on the left. Slight proptosis was present. The optic nerve head was swollen.

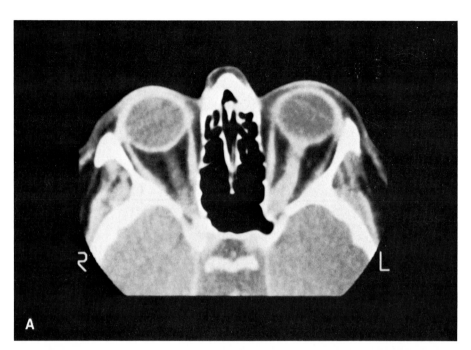

Figure A. CT with contrast demonstrates a tubular expansion of the entire intraorbital optic nerve. Enhancement is quite marked.

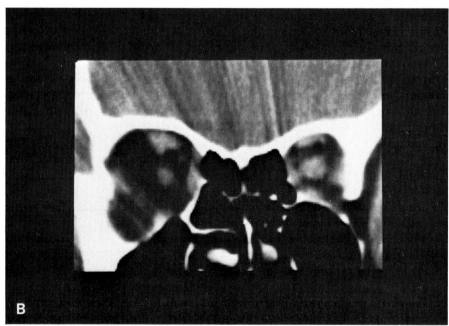

Figure B. Coronal CT confirms the enlarged left optic nerve. The central lucency represents the optic nerve, which is surrounded by the denser optic nerve sheath meningioma.

Follow-up: The patient underwent a frontotemporal craniotomy with unroofing of the optic canal. The optic nerve was excised from the globe to the chiasm. The optic nerve sheath meningioma did not extend beyond the intraorbital end of the optic canal.

CASE 21. Optic Nerve Sheath Meningioma

This 41-year-old female presented with 3-year history of blurred vision and right-sided proptosis. Visual acuity: 20/20 OU. The right eye was 2.5 mm more prominent than the left. Fluorescein angiogram was negative. Her symptoms of blurred vision resolved. Serial CT examinations over the past 2 years have been unchanged.

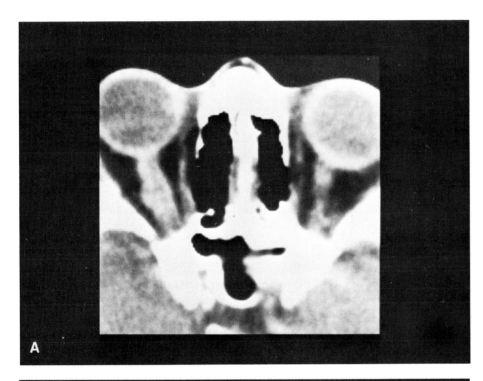

Figure A. Axial CT demonstrates tubular thickening of the right optic nerve with a "railroad" configuration, i.e., dense periphery with central lucency. Mild proptosis is evident.

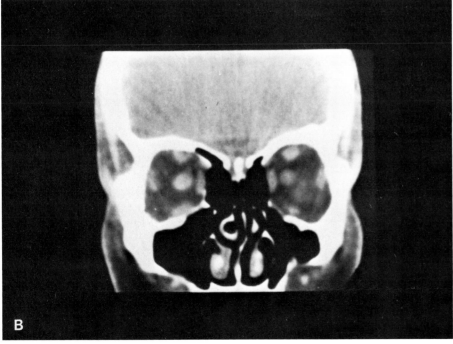

Figure B. Coronal CT reveals thickened right optic nerve with central lucency representing the entrapped optic nerve, surrounded by the denser optic nerve sheath meningioma (no histologic confirmation).

CASE 22. Optic Nerve Sheath Meningioma

A 54-year-old male with intermittent blurring of right eye for six months. Episodes increased to 7 to 10 times per day. Visual acuity at initial examination: 20/20 OU. A right lower visual field defect was present. Examination four months later revealed no light perception on the right. 20/20 OS. Fundoscopy revealed the right disc to be elevated with a blurred margin.

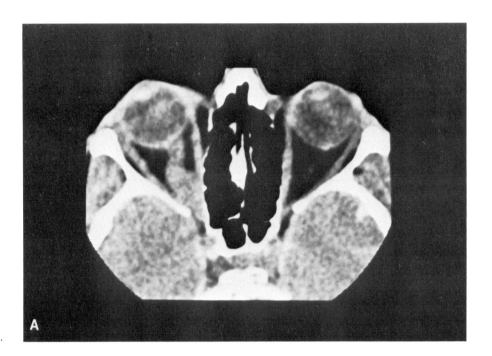

Figure A. CT demonstrates a tubular expansion of the entire right intraorbital optic nerve, especially at the orbital apex. The nerve is tortuous. Mild proptosis is present.

Follow-up: Surgical exploration via a frontal craniotomy revealed an optic nerve sheath meningioma extending beyond the intracranial end of the canal for about 4 mm. The optic chiasm was free of tumor. The optic nerve was resected from the globe to the chiasm. It was adherent to the annulus of Zinn but was thought to be completely excised.

CASE 23. Optic Nerve Sheath Meningioma

A 34-year-old male with history of having a right optic neuropathy diagnosed 10 years previously, with decreased vision. Nine years previously vision was 20/20 OD, 20/15 OS. Impaired color vision was present. Gradually lost all vision on the right. Fundoscopy did not reveal any abnormal vessels or disc atrophy.

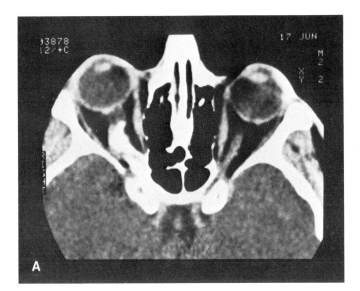

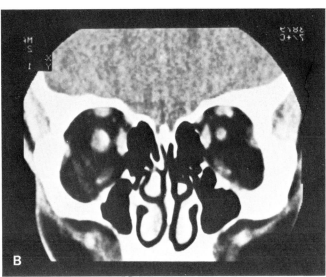

Figure A. Axial CT demonstrates diffusely thickened, tubular-shaped right optic nerve. There is dense calcium present along the nerve.

Figure B. Coronal CT demonstrates the thickened right optic nerve. The calcium is localized to the superomedial aspect of the nerve, with a lucent component immediately lateral to the calcium. This lucency probably represents the nerve itself.

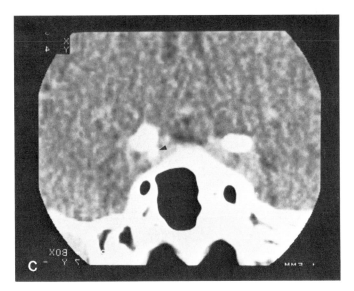

Figure C. Coronal CT at the level of the anterior clinoid processes. The calcium extends into the right optic canal (arrowhead).

Diagnosis: Optic nerve sheath meningioma (no histologic confirmation).

CASE 24. Optic Nerve Sheath Meningioma with Intracanalicular Involvement

This 68-year-old female diagnosed 4 years previously to have optic nerve sheath meningioma. Her presenting symptoms were progressive blurred vision and exophthalmos. Partial excision was achieved via a lateral orbitotomy. A second exploration via a frontal craniotomy revealed that the optic nerve sheath tumor had extended into the optic canal, with a large mass surrounding the intraorbital optic nerve. A subtotal resection was performed. On her current admission there was no light perception on the left. Cilioretinal shunt vessels were present.

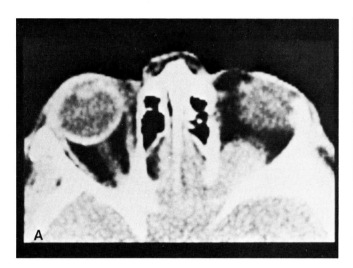

Figure A. CT demonstrating left fusiform orbital mass extending into the optic canal. The canal is considerably widened.

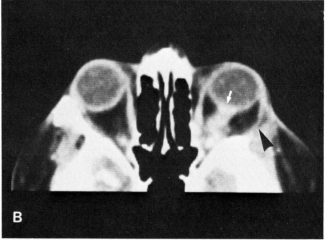

Figure B. Postoperative CT after subtotal resection of the optic nerve sheath meningioma. There is absent bone from the lateral orbitotomy (arrowhead). The entire left optic nerve is thickened with a fusiform expansion of the posterior aspect. The tumor enhances with contrast. Tumor can be visualized, extending right up to the optic nerve head (arrow).

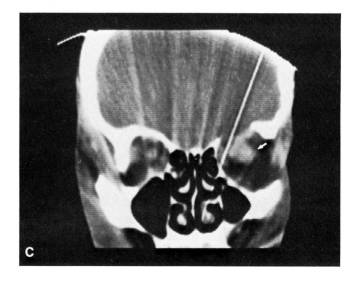

Figure C. Coronal CT (artifact lines from dental fillings) demonstrating surgical defects from the lateral orbitotomy and frontal craniotomy. The optic nerve sheath meningioma (arrow) has an irregular margin, probably related to the previous subtotal resection.

CASE 25. Optic Nerve Sheath Meningioma

A 53-year-old female with progressive loss of right temporal visual field and decreased visual acuity. Fundoscopy revealed right optic atrophy and the presence of opticocilliary shunt vessels.

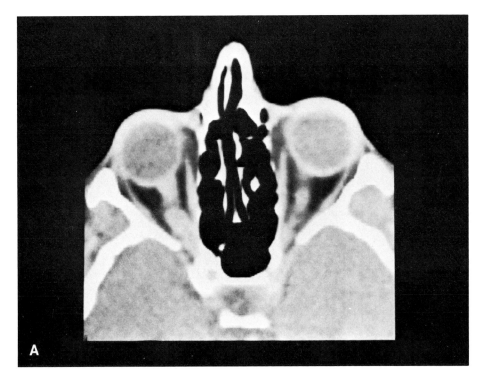

Figure A. The right optic nerve is uniformly thickened and tortuous. The nerve has enhanced to a moderate degree with contrast administration.

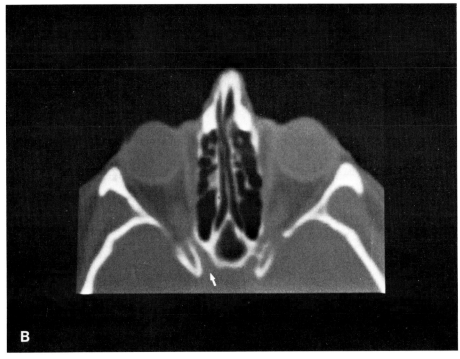

Figure B. CT of the optic canals with bone windows. The right optic canal (arrow) is enlarged with a scalloped appearance along the posterior ethmoid and sphenoid margin of the canal. There may be minimal hyperostosis along this medial margin of the canal when compared to the contralateral side.

Follow-up: Exploration via a frontal craniotomy revealed an optic nerve mass extending beyond the intracranial end of the optic canal and spreading along the adjacent dural reflections. Biopsy confirmed optic nerve sheath meningioma.

CASE 26. Optic Nerve Sheath Meningioma and Thyroid Ophthalmopathy
A 26-year-old male with Down's syndrome with loss of vision on the right for several months. Patient has been on thyroid replacement therapy. He has been clinically thyrotoxic for eight months.

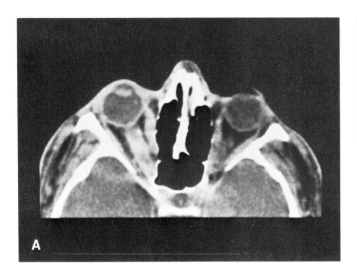 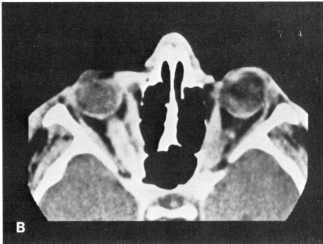

Figures A and B. The characteristic findings for an optic nerve sheath meningioma are present on the right, with a tubular expansion of the optic nerve, prominent contrast enhancement, and a linear central lucency representing the entrapped optic nerve. In addition, there is marked thickening of both medial rectus muscles secondary to the thyroid ophthalmopathy.

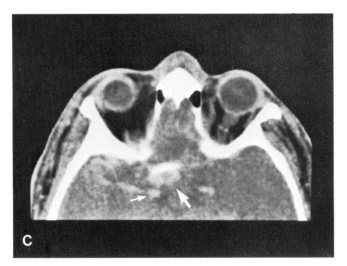 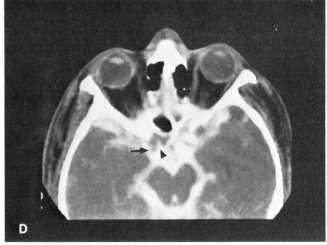

Figure C. The intracranial extent of the optic nerve sheath meningioma is visualized as an enhancing soft-tissue mass (large arrow) in the suprasellar cistern, anterior to the right internal carotid artery (small arrow).

Figure D. Metrizamide CT cisternogram clearly defines the limits of the meningioma (arrowhead) as it extends from the intracranial end of the optic canal into the suprasellar cistern, anterior to and separate from the internal carotid artery (arrow).

Follow-up: Surgery via a right orbitotomy and craniotomy revealed an optic nerve sheath meningioma that had extended intracranially beyond the optic canal, surrounding but not involving the internal carotid artery and cavernous sinus. The meningioma extended as far back as the chiasm. Resection from behind the globe to include the intracranial component was achieved.

CASE 27. Apical Meningioma
A 35-year-old male with decreased vision on the right.

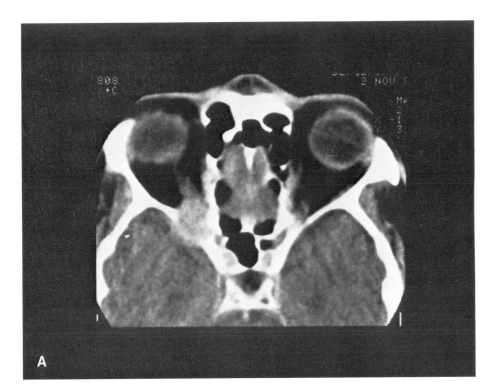

Figure A. Homogeneously enhancing mass in the orbital apex. There is destruction of the sphenoid wing and erosion of the superior orbital fissure. The mass bulges into the middle cranial fossa.

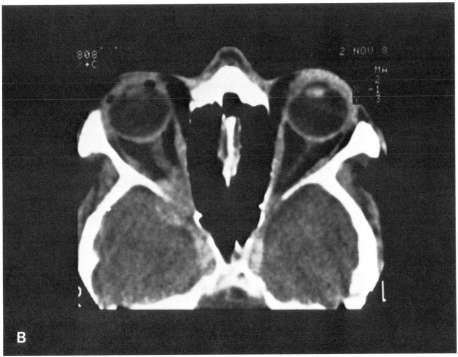

Figure B. The tumor in the orbital apex has displaced the optic nerve medially. The optic nerve is slightly thickened.

Follow-up: Surgery revealed a meningioma, probably arising from the sphenoid wing. The tumor had extended along optic nerve.

CASE 28. Optic Atrophy

A 3-year-old female with deteriorating vision, nystagmus, and seizure. Visual acuity: 20/20 OU. Both disks were pale, right greater than left. Prominent nystagmus in all directions. The visual evoked potential studies were abnormal.

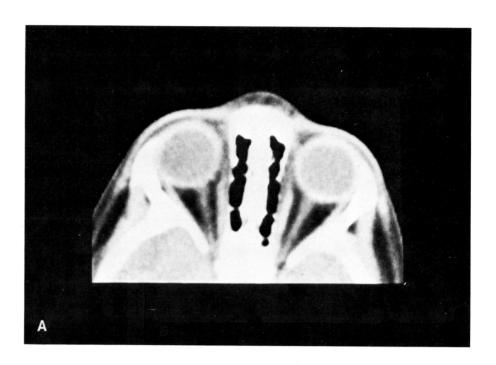

Figure A. Both optic nerves appear smaller than normal, especially on the right side, consistent with optic atrophy.

CASE 29. Familial Optic Atrophy

A 24-year-old male with progressive loss of vision since age 6 years. Appropriate family history of optic atrophy.

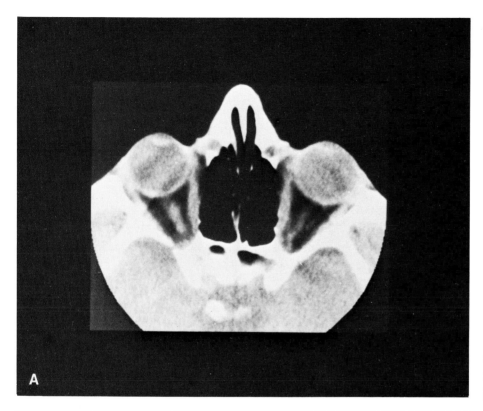

Figure A. The left optic nerve is much thinner than the normal appearing right nerve.

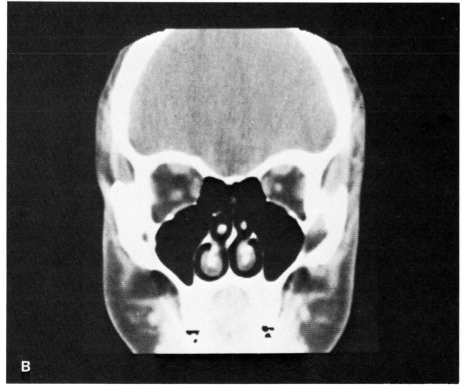

Figure B. Coronal CT confirms the reduced size of the left optic nerve.

CASE 30. Osteopetrosis with Underdevelopment of Optic Nerves

A 6-week-old male with severe congenital osteopetrosis. The electroretinogram and the cortical visual evoked potentials were markedly abnormal, indicating probable complete blindness.

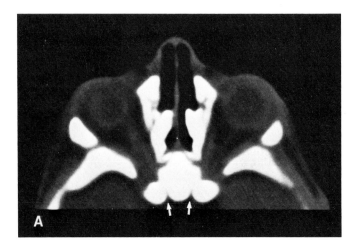

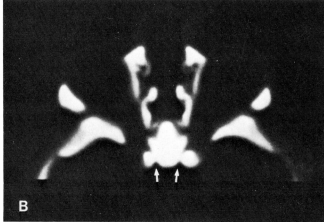

Figures A and B. CT with bone windows. All the bones are thickened and markedly sclerotic. This is particularly notable at the ethmoid laminae, which normally should be very thin. The optic canals (arrows) appear narrow due to bony overgrowth.

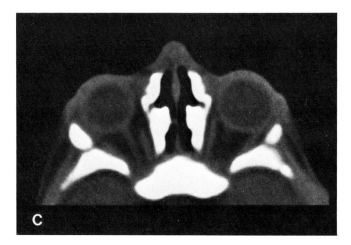

Figure C. Both optic nerves are identified. They have a thin attenuated appearance, suggesting underdevelopment.

Diagnosis: Osteopetrosis (confirmed with biopsy of extremity) with hypotrophic optic nerves, presumably secondary to constriction by the narrowed optic canals.

CASE 31. Optic Neuritis
This 10-year-old female with three-week history of pain localized to the left eye, awoke blind in the left eye one day prior to admission. Visual acuity: 20/20 OD; only light perception on the left. Fundoscopy: Papilledematous left disc; mildly abnormal right disc. Bilateral corticospinal and spinothalamic tract lesions localized to the midthoracic spinal cord were found. The findings were consistent with a demyelinating process. The presence of optic neuritis and a transverse myelitis was consistent with neuromyelitis optica (Devic's syndrome).

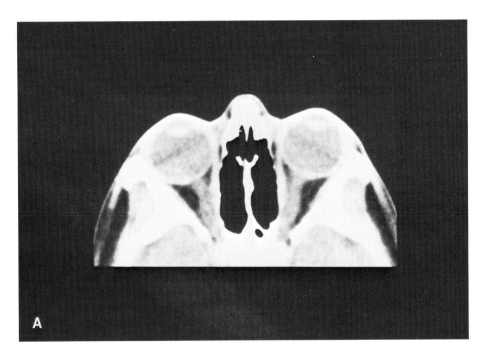

Figure A. CT demonstrates symmetrical thickening of the optic nerves due to swelling. The nerves appear somewhat inhomogeneous in density, with margins that are less well defined when compared to the configurations seen in tumors.

Follow-up: The patient was treated with steroids, and examination several months later revealed 20/20 vision bilaterally, with sharp optic discs. The other neurologic deficits had also resolved.

CASE 32. Papilledema Secondary to Benign Intracranial Hypertension
A 50-year-old female with 9-month history of headaches and blurred vision. Vision: OD 20/20, OS 20/70. Informal visual field testing suggested a bitemporal hemianopsia.

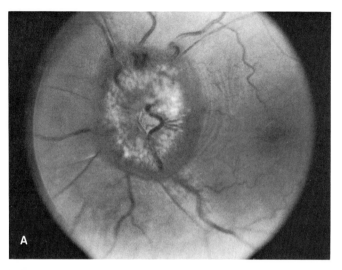
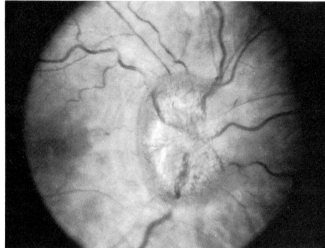

Figure A. (Left and right) Marked bilateral papilledema.

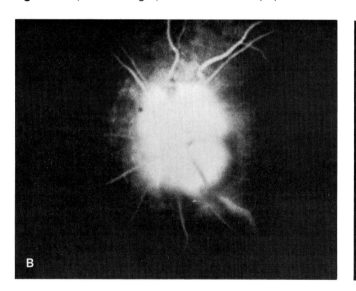
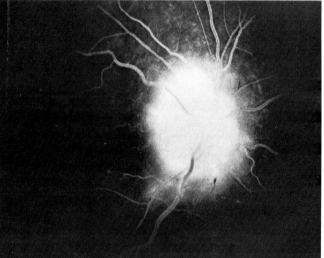

Figure B. (Left and right) Fluorescein angiogram demonstrates leakage of dye from both discs consistent with papilledema.

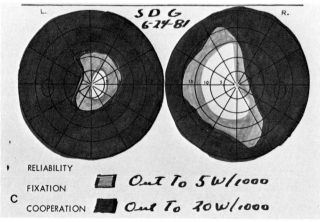

Figure C. Visual field examination reveals constricted fields with large blind spots, accounting for the bitemporal field loss.

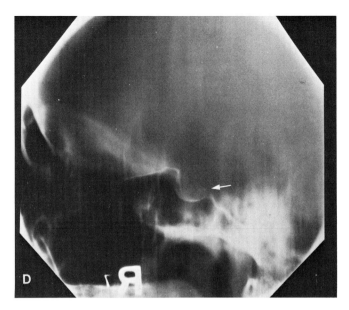

Figure D. Lateral tomogram shows a deformed sella with the dorsum amputated (arrow).

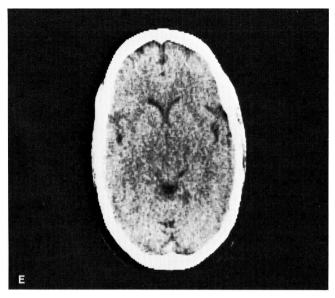

Figure E. CT of brain reveals reduced venticular size for a patient of this age.

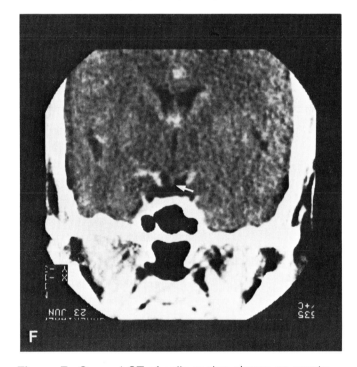

Figure F. Coronal CT of sella region shows an empty sella. The internal carotid arteries are seen laterally. The infundibular stalk (arrow) descends into the empty sella. No perisellar mass to account for the eroded dorsum is present.

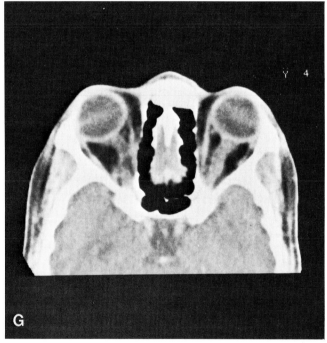

Figure G. CT of the orbits demonstrates marked bilateral optic nerve thickening consistent with papilledema. The nerves have mottled appearance.

Clinical illustrations A, B, C, I, and J courtesy of Donald Bienfang, MD.					***continued***

Figure H. CT of the optic canals demonstrates minimal enlargement of the intracranial end of the left optic canal (arrow). A lumbar puncture was performed, which revealed an opening pressure of greater than 700 mm H_2O. A diagnosis of pseudotumor cerebri (benign intracranial hypertension) was made. The small ventricles, erosive bone changes of the dorsum sella, the empty sella, the enlargement of the left optic canal, and papilledema could all be accounted for on the basis of chronic increased intracranial pressure. The patient was treated with multiple lumbar punctures, steroids, and diuretics. The CSF pressure decreased to 150 mm H_2O.

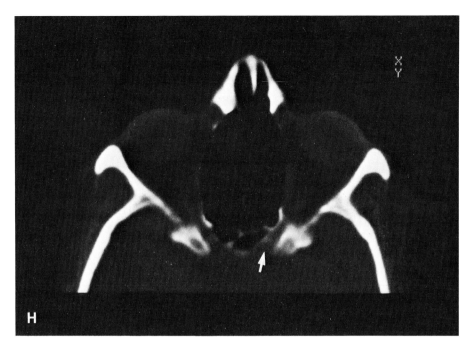

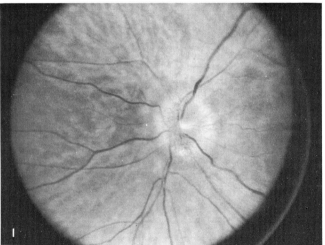 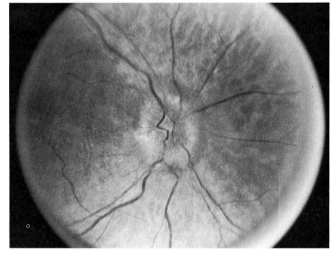

Figure I. (Left and right) Follow-up fundoscopy at three weeks. Vision: 20/20 OD, 20/80 OS. There is reduced swelling of the optic discs.

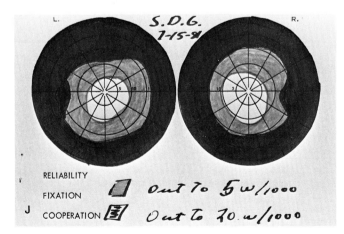 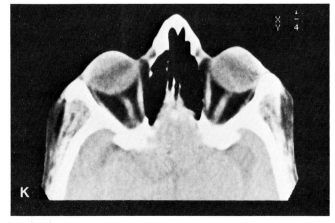

Figure J. Visual fields reveal return of central vision.

Figure K. Follow-up CT scan of orbits shows marked reduction in the size of the optic nerves, which now appear smaller than normal and suggest optic atrophy.

CHAPTER FOUR

Primary Orbital Neoplasms

Three different embryonic layers, the neural ectoderm, surface ectoderm, and mesoderm participate in development of the orbit and its contents. As a result, the orbit contains many different types of tissue—including bone, muscle, fat, nerves, skin, and glandular tissue. Therefore, it is not surprising that the orbit can be involved in a wide spectrum of a neoplastic diseases. Specific tumors are more likely to occur in certain parts of the orbit. Exophthalmos is by far the most common presenting sign of orbital tumors and is a relatively nonspecific sign. Nevertheless, tumors arising in certain parts of the orbit may have a special complex of symptoms peculiar to that orbital site. For these reasons, as well as for surgical planning, it is convenient to divide the orbit into various compartments.

Ocular lesions present with blurred vision and increasing scotomata due to retinal detachment. Tumors of the anterior orbit, including the lids and conjunctiva, cause local irritation and mass effect that are usually clinically apparent by visual inspection. Ocular lesions are discussed in Chapter 8.

The retrobulbar space is that part of the orbit posterior to the globe and orbital septum. It is bounded by the bony orbit and is divided into the intraconal and extraconal spaces. The intraconal space includes the optic nerve and its surrounding sheath, which are discussed in Chapter 3. Other primary neoplasms of the intraconal and extraconal spaces are the subject of this chapter. Lesions of the bony orbit, paranasal sinuses, intracranial cavity, and metastatic disease can involve the orbit secondarily, and these are discussed separately in Chapter 5.

Although exophthalmos is the most common presenting sign, retrobulbar lesions can be associated with pain and periorbital edema. Furthermore, progressive visual impairment may result from pressure on or stretching of the optic nerve. If the retrobulbar tumor extends into the orbital apex or superior orbital fissure, the patient may develop an opthalmoplegia.[1]

In the CT evaluation of orbital tumors, the amount of proptosis can be assessed by the techniques suggested by Hilal and Trokel.[2] Using a midorbital axial scan, a straight line is drawn between the anterior margins of the zygomatic processes. The distance between the anterior cornea and the interzygomatic line is normally 21 mm or less. It is important that the scan be through the midaxial plane of the orbit.

After assessing proptosis, identify the mass and measure its size. Define the surface characteristics of the mass. Are the margins smooth, lobulated, or irregular? These features help determine whether it is a benign, well-encapsulated mass or a poorly defined, infiltrating malignant lesion. Does it displace normal structures or invade them? Next, note the internal character of the tumor to see if it is homogeneous or heterogeneous. Also, determine the density or absorption values on the plain scan and the amount of contrast enhancement. Does the entire mass enhance or is there a necrotic center? Finally, look at the bony orbit to identify any bone extension, bone erosion, or hyperostosis.[3–6]

For surgical planning and to determine resectability, it is essential to define the location and extent of the tumor. As mentioned earlier, it is helpful to place the mass in a particular compartment of the orbit. The relationship of the optic nerve to the mass is critical in deciding whether or not it can be removed with a lateral Kronlein orbitotomy. If the nerve is stretched around the lateral aspect of the mass, a medial approach may be necessary. Involvement of the orbital apex may require unroofing of the orbit to accomplish a complete resection. Finally, the CT scan is helpful to evaluate any extraorbital extension, particularly extension through the superior orbital fissure into intracranial compartments.

With all this information obtained from the CT scan, it is possible in many cases to predict the histopathology of the lesion. At least, a limited differential can be determined to assist in therapeutic planning.

VASCULAR NEOPLASMS

Vascular neoplasms represent 10 to 15 percent of all orbital tumors. The majority of these are cavernous hemangioma and lymphangioma.

Cavernous Hemangioma *(Cases 1–3)*

Cavernous hemangiomas are one of the more common orbital tumors in the adult, presenting in the second to the fourth decade. They grow slowly but do not involute. Accelerated growth has been observed during pregnancy. They are benign, well-encapsulated lesions with wide vascular spaces.[7] Although vascular, cavernous hemangiomas are somehow isolated from the arterial circulation of the orbit. They are characterized by slow intratumor circulation, feeding arteries of small caliber and a few dilated veins. Often no blush is present on the arteriogram, although small angiomatous spots may be seen with subtraction angiography.[8] Cavernous hemangiomas may be partially thrombosed and occasionally calcify.

CT Findings: Cavernous hemangiomas are high-absorption lesions on plain scan and demonstrate marked homogeneous contrast enhancement. They have smooth, well-defined margins and are round or oval in shape.[5,9] In Davis et al.'s series of 18 cases,[10] 83 percent were intraconal, and 17 of 18 were primarily retrobulbar in location. Two-thirds were lateral to the optic nerve, either superior or inferior. All but one case showed expansion of the bony orbit, indicative of a slow-growing, benign lesion that has been present for many years. Occasionally, a cavernous hemangioma may involve the orbital apex. Wende et al.,[3] reported similar findings in another 18 cases of cavernous hemangioma.

Lymphangioma *(Cases 4 and 5)*

Lymphangiomas consist of bloodless channels that resemble lymphatics surrounded by lymphoid tissue. Since normally no lymphatic tissue exists in the orbit, these tumors probably arise from an anlage of vascular mesenchyme capable of lymphatic differentiation. Retrobulbar tumors may be associated with similar lesions on the conjunctiva and lids.[1]

Lymphangiomas occur in children and young adults. They are slowly progressive and do not spontaneously regress. Although benign, they do not have a capsule, and they infiltrate orbital tissue, making surgical resection very difficult and sometimes futile. Increased exophthalmos is often associated with upper respiratory tract infections due to hyperplasia of the lymphoid tissue in the tumor. Intratumoral hemorrhage is another feature that can result in sudden increased proptosis. The hematoma has been called a "blood cyst" or "chocolate cyst," depending on whether the blood is fresh or old.[7] Lloyd[11] reported four cases of blood cysts associated with acute proptosis and loss of vision.

CT Findings. Lymphangiomas are high-absorption lesions on plain scan but are also characteristically heterogeneous, having areas within the tumor of varying density. They usually show little or no contrast enhancement. Their margins are irregular and poorly defined. In their series of seven cases, Davis et al.[10] observed other features that were helpful in distinguishing lymphangioma from hemangioma. Most lymphangiomas were extraconal, but some involved both compartments of the retrobulbar space. Lymphangiomas were equally likely to be found anterior or posterior to the globe or even diffusely. The majority were medial to the optic nerve. Since lymphangiomas are also characterized by slow, relentless growth, expansion of the bony orbit can occur.

Capillary Hemangioma *(Case 6)*

Capillary hemangiomas, also called benign hemangioendothelioma or strawberry hemangioma of childhood, occur in the first year of life. They grow for about six months and then tend to involute spontaneously.[7] They may present as a raised and red lesion (strawberry nevus) on an eyelid or may be part of a larger superficial facial lesion. In either case, the orbital involvement is often more extensive than is suspected clinically. Unlike cavernous hemangioma, they are highly vascular and can receive prominent vascular supply from the ophthalmic artery and multiple branches of the external carotid artery.[8]

Hemangiopericytoma *(Case 7)*

Hemangiopericytomas are slow-growing vascular tumors and usually have a capsule. Nevertheless, they are locally aggressive and can destroy bone to extend beyond the orbit. Metastases can also occur. A dense homogeneous stain is usually seen angiographically.[12]

CT Findings: Hemangiopericytomas usually appear encapsulated and well defined, more often occurring in the intraconal space. They are high-absorption areas on plain scan and enhance. In Cromwell et al.'s report of two cases,[12] both lesions were very dense on both the plain and contrast scan.

TUMORS IN CHILDREN

In addition to lymphangioma and capillary hemangioma, other tumors that occur primarily in childhood include rhabdomyosarcoma, teratoma, optic nerve glioma and retinoblastoma. Optic nerve gliomas and retinoblastomas are discussed in Chapters 3 and 8, respectively.

Rhabdomyosarcoma (Cases 8–10)

Embryonal rhabdomyosarcoma is the most common primary malignant orbital tumor of childhood. It is a primitive malignant tumor that arises from embryonic mesenchyme within orbital soft tissue rather than from the extraocular muscles. These tumors usually present with rapid progressive exophthalmos. They are aggressive, and if not diagnosed and treated promptly, they destroy the bony orbit and extend beyond the orbit.[13]

CT Findings. Rhabdomyosarcoma arises in the retrobulbar compartment and by the time of presentation usually involves both the intraconal and extraconal spaces. They are of average density on plain scan and show mild to moderate contrast enhancement. The CT scan is most helpful to evaluate extension into the orbital apex and extraorbital involvement.[14]

Teratomas (Case 11)

Teratomas are usually present at birth or appear in the first few months of life. They are benign but can be very large, causing gross enlargement of the orbit and distortion of the normal orbital structures. Teratomas contain multiple tissues from all three germ layers.[15,16]

CT Findings. Since teratomas contain many different tissues, they often have a heterogeneous appearance on CT scan. Areas of calcification or fat density may be seen. If cystic components are identified, aspiration may relieve some of the pressure and mass effect. CT shows the relationship of the tumor to the normal soft-tissue structures of the orbit, as well as the character and degree of deformity of the bony orbit.

OTHER SOLID AND CYSTIC LESIONS

Lymphoma (Cases 12–19)

A better understanding of lymphomatous tumors has been heralded by two new developments. First, many lesions previously called lymphoma have been redefined as reactive hyperplasia (pseudotumors) composed of mature lymphocytes. Second, lymphomas have been reclassified based on immunopathology, whereby the lymphoreticular cells have been subdivided into B- and T-lymphocytes and M-cells.[17] Most lymphomas and lymphatic leukemias are derangements of the B-cell line. Hodgkin's disease is a derangement of the T-cell line, and M-cell line is represented by true histiocytic lesions, such as the reticuloendothelioses and histiocytoses.[17,18]

Small collections of lymphoid tissue are found normally in the conjunctiva and lacrimal gland. The rest of the orbit has very little lymphoid tissue. Primary orbital lymphoma is unusual. There are often subclinical extraorbital sites that become apparent later in the course of the disease. Pseudotumor may be a precursor of primary orbital lymphoma. The incidence of systemic lymphomatous involvement of the orbit is about 3.3 percent, with the conjunctiva being involved three times more often than other orbital sites. Orbital lymphoma may present with lid swelling and edema or proptosis, depending on whether it arises in the anterior orbit or retrobulbar space, respectively.[19]

CT Findings: Lymphomas are homogeneous-appearing lesions found in the anterior orbit or the extraconal space of the retrobulbar compartment. The retrobulbar lesions are usually fairly well delineated by the orbital fat, but if they are adjacent to the orbital septum, they may be more ill-defined surrounding the sclera of the globe. They are of average density on plain scan and show mild to moderate enhancement.[2,4,20]

Neurofibroma–Neurilemoma (Cases 20–22)

Both neurofibroma and neurilemoma are slow-growing peripheral-nerve tumors. They present in middle age and are located in the retrobulbar compartment. Neurilemomas (schwannomas) arise from the Schwann cell and are encapsulated by perineural cells. They often compress the adjacent nerve origin, causing pain. Neurofibromas contain Schwann cells, endoneural cells, and axons. They are not encapsulated but may be well circumscribed. The nerve of origin is frequently difficult to identify. Unlike neurilemoma, neurofibromas are usually painless. Neurofibromas are twice as common as neurilemomas. If a neurofibroma is associated with neurofibromatosis, it is usually more extensive and likely to recur after surgical resection. In addition, there is a 10 percent chance of malignant transformation of these neurofibromas.[21]

CT Findings. Neurofibromas and neurilemomas can be found in the extraconal or intraconal spaces. They have well-defined margins, although the margins may have a lobulated contour. They are usually of average density on plain scan and demonstrate moderate to marked homogeneous contrast enhancement.[2,4]

Fibrous Histiocytoma (Fibroxanthoma)

Fibrous histiocytomas combine features of the fibroblast and histiocyte. Most are benign, but they are not encapsulated and are locally infiltrative.[22] These tumors are vascular, and the angiogram characteristically shows a dense homogeneous stain.[23]

CT Findings. Fibrous histiocytomas usually have well-defined margins and can be found in the intraconal or extraconal compartments or both. They are homogeneous and of average density on plain scan and show moderate to marked contrast enhancement.

Dermoid Cyst *(Cases 23–27)*

Dermoid cysts arise from epithelial rests of cells found at sutural sites where surface ectoderm is pinched off during the development of the orbital bones. They are most commonly found along the superotemporal orbital rim and therefore enter into the differential diagnosis of lacrimal gland tumors. They are often attached to the orbital bones. The cystic center contains epithelial debris.[15]

CT Findings. Dermoid cysts have a characteristic appearance on CT scan. The margins are smooth and clearly defined, and the cystic center occupies most of the tumor volume.[24] The cystic center is almost always of low absorption, occasionally approaching minus 100 units.[3] The rim of the cyst may enhance with contrast. Many dermoid cysts cause benign bone expansion of the lateral and superior orbital walls.[25]

LACRIMAL GLAND TUMORS

The lacrimal gland is located in the superior lateral aspect of the orbit, adjacent to the tendons of the superior and lateral rectus muscles. It bridges the orbital septum in an extraconal position (see Chapter 1). Similar to the salivary glands histologically, the lacrimal gland is involved by similar disease processes. Epithelial tumors represent 50 percent of lacrimal gland mass lesions. Half of these are pleomorphic adenomas, and the other half are in a malignant category, which includes adenocystic, pleomorphic, mucoepidermoid, adenocarcinoma, and squamous cell and undifferentiated carcinoma. The remaining 50 percent of lacrimal gland masses are of the lymphoid-inflammatory type, which represents a spectrum from benign dacryoadenitis to malignant lymphoma.[26,27] Lacrimal gland tumors present clinically with fullness of the eyelid, ptosis, or unilateral exophthalmos. Pressure on the globe may cause double vision.

Pleomorphic Adenoma
(Benign Mixed Adenoma) *(Cases 28 and 29)*

Pleomorphic adenomas are the most common tumors of the lacrimal gland. They are slow growing and well encapsulated. They may have small cystic areas within them. Microcalcifications are often seen pathologically.[26]

CT Findings. Pleomorphic adenomas have a variable appearance on CT scan. They are high-absorption lesions on plain scan and enhance moderately with contrast. Those with cystic components appear more heterogeneous and may not enhance. The tumor margins are smooth and well defined. The smaller lesions are found in the region of the lacrimal fossa and displace the globe medially and inferiorly. As they enlarge they extend posteriorly along the extraconal space, displacing the muscle cone and optic nerve medially and the globe anteriorly. Although pleomorphic adenomas are not locally invasive, they often induce some local bone reaction or erosion. Occasionally, they actually may be imbedded in the orbital wall.[24]

Adenocystic Carcinoma *(Case 30)*

Adenocystic carcinomas are the most common malignant tumors of the lacrimal gland; they are infiltrating lesions and readily destroy bone, frequently extend posteriorly into the orbital apex, and have a tendency to extend along nerves to cause pain early in the course of the disease. Pain is a common symptom with adenocystic carcinoma as opposed to other orbital tumors.[27]

CT Findings. Adenocystic carcinomas have irregular, poorly defined margins. They often extend posteriorly along the extraconal space to infiltrate other retrobulbar orbital structures. Destruction of the lateral wall is often seen, with tumor extending into the temporal fossa, orbital apex, or even the middle cranial fossa. These tumors are usually of average absorption on plain scan and show moderate contrast enhancement.[3,4]

Adenocarcinoma *(Case 31)*

Adenocarcinomas of the lacrimal gland are much less common. They are also malignant and aggressive and have a poor prognosis.

CT Findings. The CT appearance of adenocarcinoma is essentially indistinguishable from adenocystic carcinoma. The adenocarcinoma in our series did not enhance[24]; however, Gyldensted et al.[4] reported a case that showed profound enhancement.

Mucoepidermoid Carcinoma–Pleomorphic (Malignant Mixed) Carcinoma

Both of these tumors are malignant and infiltrating lesions. In our series of 11 cases of lacrimal gland tumors,[24] there were three mucoepidermoid carcinomas but no pleomorphic carcinomas. Pleomorphic carcinoma represents malignant degeneration of a pleomorphic adenoma. A significant number of other malignant tumors of the lacrimal gland probably also arise within pleomorphic adenomas. Some pathologists classify all such lesions as pleomorphic carcinomas; our pathologists classify them according to the predominant cell type. Therefore, our cases of mucoepidermoid carcinoma might be classified as pleomorphic carcinomas by other pathologists.

CT Findings. Our mucoepidermoid carcinomas were of high absorption on plain scan and demonstrated marked contrast enhancement. The margins were moderately well defined compared to other malignant lesions.[24] These tumors can erode bone or even induce hyperostosis and thickening of the orbital wall.

Lymphoid-Inflammatory Group (Cases 32–34)

It can be very difficult to differentiate pathologically benign lymphocytic infiltration and lymphoid hyperplasia from lymphoma. Sometimes a patient needs to be followed clinically in order to determine the true nature of the disease. Lymphocytic infiltration of the lacrimal gland occurs in Sjögren's syndrome. Mikulicz syndrome is a nonspecific swelling of the lacrimal and salivary glands, associated with conditions such as leukemia, lymphosarcoma, tuberculosis, syphilis, and sarcoidosis.[26,27]

CT Findings. One or both lacrimal glands may be involved by the lymphoid-inflammatory group of diseases. These lesions have a variable appearance on CT scan. Most have well-defined margins and a homogeneous appearance. In our series of five cases[24] there was moderate enhancement in Sjögren's and Mikulicz syndromes but only mild enhancement in lymphoid hyperplasia.

Miscellaneous Tumors (Cases 35–41)

Aside from fibrous histiocytoma, tumors of fibrous origin are uncommon. Fibrosarcomas are malignant and usually arise years after radiotherapy. Takahashi and Tamakawa[28] reported a case that, surprisingly, was fairly well defined. It enhanced moderately with contrast material. Gyldensted et al.[4] reported a case that showed only minimal enhancement.

Except for rhabdomyosarcoma, mesenchymal tumors—such as leiomyoma, leiomyosarcoma, lipoma, and liposarcoma—are also rare in the orbit. Takahashi and Tamakawa[28] also reported a mesenchymoma that was intraconal, poorly defined, and of slightly increased density on CT scan.

Primary bone and cartilagenous tumors can arise within the bony orbit and encroach on orbital structures. Osteomas usually arise within the frontal and ethmoid sinuses and involve the orbit secondarily. Osteosarcoma, chondroma, and chondrosarcoma are rare, but when they occur, their radiographic features are similar to those seen in other bones of the body. Fibrous dysplasia is not a true tumor. The exuberant fibro-osseous material associated with this disease often encroaches on the orbital space and causes proptosis.[22] Metastases can occur to the bony orbit, as discussed in Chapter 5.

REFERENCES

1. Jones IS, Jakobiec FA, Nolan B: Patient examination and introduction to orbital disease. In Jones IS, Jakobiec FA (eds): Diseases of the Orbit. Hagerstown, Md., Harper & Row, Chap 1, 1979, pp 1–30
2. Hilal SK, Trokel SL: Computerized tomography of the orbit using thin sections. Semin Roentgenol 12:137–147, 1977
3. Wende S, Aulich A, Nover A, et al: Computed tomography of orbital lesions. A cooperative study of 210 cases. Neuroradiology 13:123–134, 1977
4. Gyldensted C, Lester J, Fledelius H: Computed tomography of orbital lesions. A radiological study of 144 cases. Neuroradiology 13:141–150, 1977
5. Forbes GS, Sheedy PF II, Waller RR: Orbital tumors evaluated by computed tomography. Radiology 136:101–111, 1980
6. Tadmor R, New PFJ: Computed tomography of the orbit with special emphasis on coronal sections: Part II. Pathological anatomy. J Comput Assist Tomogr 2:35–44, 1978
7. Jakobiec FA, Jones IS: Vascular tumors, malformations and degenerations. In Jones IS, Jakobiec FA (eds): Diseases of the Orbit. Hagerstown, Md., Harper & Row, Chap 14, 1979, pp 269–308
8. Dilenge D: Arteriography in angiomas of the orbit. Radiology 113:355–361, 1974
9. Salvolini U, Menichelli F, Pasquini U: Computer assisted tomography in 90 cases of exophthalmos. J Comput Assist Tomogr 1:81–100, 1977
10. Davis KR, Hesselink JR, Dallow RL, Grove AS: CT and ultrasound in the diagnosis of cavernous hemangioma and lymphangioma of the orbit. CT 4:98–104, 1980
11. Lloyd GAS: The impact of CT scanning and ultrasonography on orbital diagnosis. Clin Radiol 28:583–593, 1977
12. Cromwell LD, Kerber C, Margolis MT: Selective carotid angiography in the diagnosis of orbital hemangiopericytoma: Report of two cases. AJR 129:730–733, 1977
13. Knowles DM II, Jakobiec FA, Jones IS: Rhabomyosarcoma. In Jones IS, Jakobiec FA (eds): Diseases of the Orbit. Hagerstown, Md., Harper & Row, Chap 19, 1979, pp 435–460
14. Zimmerman RA, Bilaniuk LT, Littman P, Raney RB: Computed tomography of pediatric craniofacial sarcoma. CT 2:113–121, 1978
15. Howard GM: Cystic tumors. In Jones IS, Jakobiec FA (eds): Diseases of the Orbit. Hagerstown, Md., Harper & Row, Chap 9, 1979, pp. 135–144
16. Barber JC, Barber LF, Guerry D, Geeraets WJ: Congenital orbital teratoma. Arch Ophthalmol 91:45–48, 1974
17. Hansen, JA, Good RA: Malignant diseases of the lymphoid system in immunological perspective. Hum Pathol 5:567–599, 1974
18. Lukes R, Collins R: Immunologic characterization of human malignant lymphoma. Cancer 34:1488–1503, 1974
19. Jakobiec FA, Jones IS: Lymphomatous, plasmacytic, histiocytic and hematopoietic tumors. In Jones IS, Jakobiec FA (eds): Diseases of the Orbit. Hagerstown, Md., Harper and Row, Chap 15, 1979, pp 309–354
20. Momose KJ, New PFJ, Grove AS, Scott WR: The use of computed tomography in ophthalmology. Radiology 115:361–368, 1975

21. Jakobiec FA, Jones IS: Neurogenic tumors. In Jones IS, Jakobiec FA (eds.): Diseases of the Orbit. Hagerstown, Md., Harper & Row, Chap 17, 1979, pp. 371–416

22. Jakobiec FA, Jones IS: Mesenchymal and fibro-osseous tumors. In Jones IS, and Jakobiec FA (eds.): Diseases of the Orbit. Hagerstown, Md., Harper & Row, Chap 20, 1979, pp 461–502.

23. Cromwell LD, Kerber C: Selective carotid angiography in the diagnosis of fibrous histiocytoma. Radiology 117:329–330, 1975

24. Hesselink JR, Davis KR, Dallow RL, Roberson GH, Taveras JM: Computed tomography of masses in the lacrimal gland region. Radiology 131:143–147, 1979

25. Wakenheim A, vanDamme W, Kosmann P, Bittighoffer B: Computed tomography in ophthalmology. Neuroradiology 13:135–138, 1977

26. Ashton N: Epithelial tumors of the lacrimal gland. Mod Probl Ophthalmol 14:306–323, 1975

27. Henderson JW: Orbital Tumors. Philadelphia, Saunders, 1973, pp 409–443

28. Takahashi M, Tamakawa Y: Coronal computed tomography in orbital disease. J Comput Assist Tomogr 1:505–509, 1977

CASE 1. Cavernous Hemangioma

This 39-year-old male had progressive left exophthalmos during the past 2 or 3 years. He had no pain and his vision was normal.

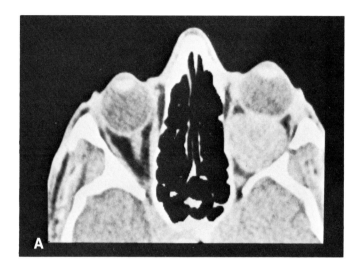

Figure A. An axial scan through the midportion of the orbits shows a large mass in the left orbit. The mass is intraconal and displaces the medial and lateral rectus muscles against the adjacent bony walls. The globe is indented posteriorly and displaced anteriorly. The left orbit is enlarged compared to the right, indicating the slow growth characteristics of the mass. It is smoothly marginated, has a homogeneous appearance, and has relatively high absorption values on this plain scan.

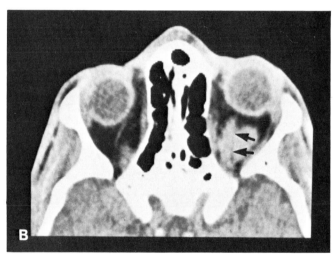

Figure B. A higher section shows the optic nerve arcing over the top of the mass (arrows).

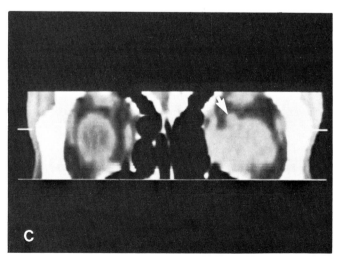

Figure C. A coronal scan confirms the position of the optic nerve over the superior medial aspect of the tumor (arrow).

Surgical Findings: At surgery a well-encapsulated mass was found that proved to be a cavernous hemangioma.

CASE 2. Cavernous Hemangioma

A 57-year-old female with right-sided exophthalmos first noted 8 years previously with progression more recently.

Clinical Findings: Vision 20/25 bilaterally. Right proptosis with increased ocular resistance. Motility normal. Ultrasound examination demonstrated a heterogeneous retrobulbar mass.

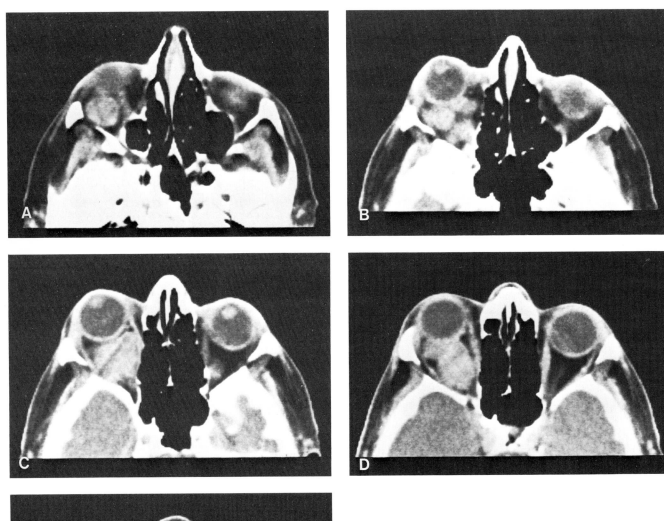

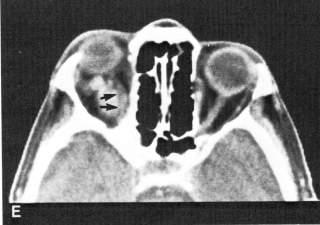

Figures A–E. Serial 5-mm CT sections with contrast. A homogeneous enhancing multilobulated but sharply marginated retrobulbar mass is demonstrated. The lesion is within the muscle cone. In Fig. C the medial rectus muscle is bowed medially. In the most craniad section, Fig. E, the optic nerve is identified displaced upwards and medially (arrows). The orbit is enlarged, with the medial wall bulging slightly into the adjacent ethmoid sinus.

Surgical Findings: Three separate encapsulated lobulated cavernous hemangiomas were removed from within the muscle cone.

CASE 3. Cavernous Hemangioma

This 50-year-old male stated that his right eye had been abnormal for several years, being teary and irritated with tunnel vision. During the past eight months his vision progressively worsened. He had recently developed right periorbital headaches and numbness of the right side of the face. He was unable to close his right eye.

Clinical Findings: Patient could only count fingers with his right eye. He had obvious proptosis and a right third nerve palsy. Ultrasonography showed an abnormality within the muscle cone posteriorly, which seemed to correspond with the optic nerve course.

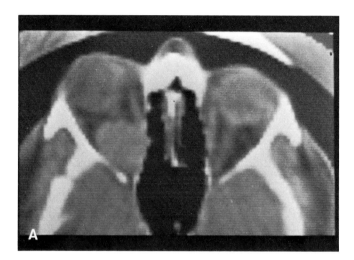 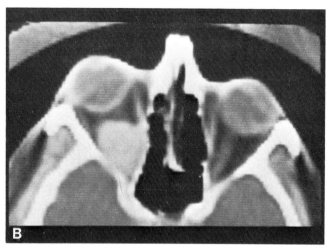

Figure A. Plain scan shows a mass in the right orbital apex. The medial rectus is displaced medially, suggesting an intraconal location. The lamina papyracea is bowed medially. The margins of the mass are slightly irregular but well defined.

Figure B. A contrast scan shows marked homogeneous contrast enhancement. The globe is proptotic.*

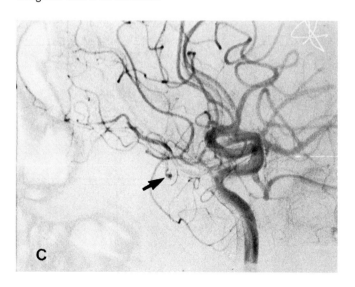

Figure C. Lateral view of a carotid arteriogram. The ophthalmic artery is displaced superiorly. The mass is relatively avascular, but there is an early-filling venous structure (arrow) that persisted into the venous phase.

Surgical Findings: With a right frontotemporal craniotomy, the roof of the orbit was removed. A 3-cm cavernous hemangioma was found in the apex of the orbit. It was adherent to the optic nerve and the nerves within the superior orbital fissure and could not be completely resected.

*Reprinted from Davis KR, Hesselink JR, Dallow RL, et al: CT and ultrasound in the diagnosis of cavernous hemangioma and lymphangioma of the orbit. CT 4(2): 101, 1980, with permission.

CASE 4. Lymphangioma
This 14-week-old female was born with a mass under her right eyebrow that extended into the upper lid. The mass was soft and compressible and caused slight ptosis. Vision was normal.

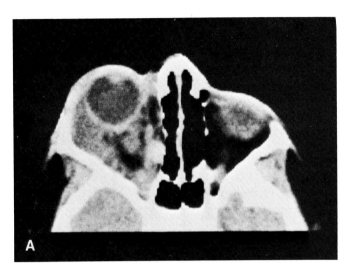

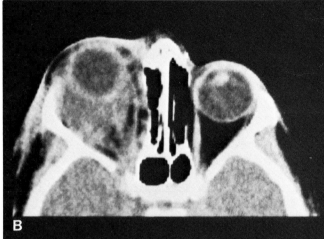

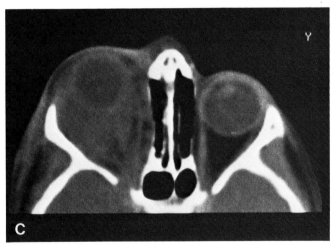

Figures A–C. Axial scans demonstrate a large mass in the right orbit, which displaces the globe anteriorly. The mass has irregular, ill-defined margins and is slightly heterogeneous. It involves both the intraconal and extraconal spaces and extends anteriorly lateral to the globe. Soft-tissue density is also seen in the orbital apex associated with widening of the superior orbital fissure. The sclerouveal rim of the globe appears thickened. The right orbit is grossly enlarged.

Diagnosis: The biopsy, performed at the age of two years, revealed a lymphangioma.

CASE 5. Lymphangioma

This nine-year-old male was normal until two years of age, when he developed slight swelling of the left upper lid. Blockage of the tear duct was suspected, but the fullness of the lid persisted, and he was referred to an ophthalmologist two to three months later. Biopsy of the lesion was followed immediately by hemorrhage, which required two aspirations. The pathologic diagnosis at that time was hemangioma. At eight years of age, trauma resulted in increased swelling of the lid, but it returned to a baseline level in three weeks. The patient was presently admitted because of increased swelling of both the upper and lower lids and because of increasing proptosis.

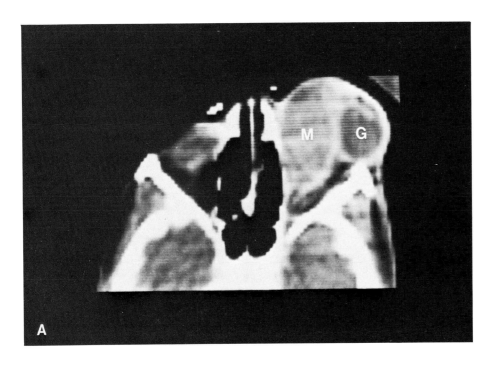

Figure A. CT scan demonstrates a large extraconal mass (M) in the medial aspect of the left orbit. The globe (G) is flattened and markedly displaced laterally. The mass has a low-density heterogeneous matrix.*

Surgical Findings: The tumor was approached through the upper lid. After aspiration of 90 ml of dark-colored fluid, the lesion was biopsied.
Final Diagnosis: Lymphangioma with an old intratumor hemorrhage.

Reprinted from Davis KR, Hesselink JR, Dallow RL, et al: CT and ultrasound in the diagnosis of cavernous hemangioma and lymphangioma of the orbit. CT 4(2): 100, 1980, with permission.

CASE 6. Capillary Hemangioma

A six-week-old infant with five-day history of intermittent swelling of the right eye. Examination revealed a markedly proptotic right eye. The periorbital area was erythematous. There was resistance to retropulsion. No bruit was detected and the fundus was normal. The left eye was normal.

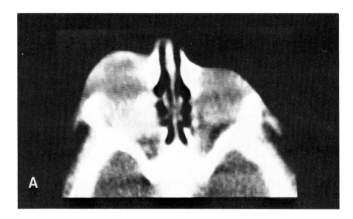 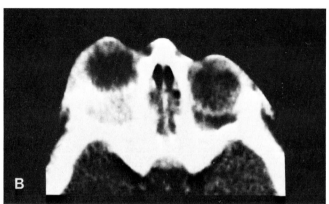

Figures A and B. Contrast-enhanced CT demonstrates marked proptosis. There is a mass that involves the entire retrobulbar space, with rather profound enhancement.

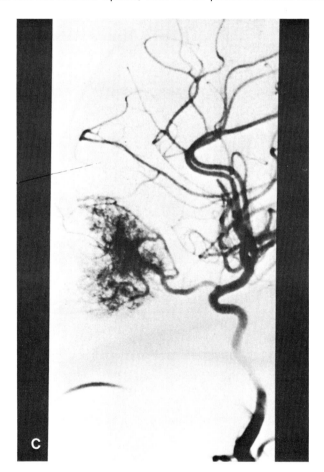 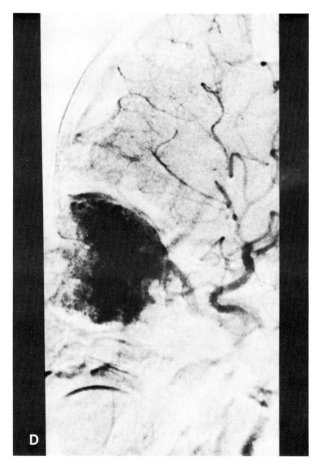

Figure C. Lateral view from a carotid arteriogram demonstrates an intense orbital vascular blush occurring in the early arterial phase. The ophthalmic artery is enlarged.

Figure D. The blush becomes more intense in the capillary phase. No arteriovenous shunting is apparent.

Follow-up: Biopsy confirmed a capillary hemangioma.

CASE 7. Hemangiopericytoma

This 44-year-old female first noted intermittent pressure and pain behind her right eye 6 years ago. Two years ago, right exophthalmos was noted and an exploration and biopsy was performed. The biopsy revealed normal ectopic lacrimal gland tissue. Recently, she noticed constant diplopia and increasing prominence of the right eye.

Clinical Findings: Vision was 20/25 OD and 20/20 OS. Proptosis of 4 mm of the right eye. Limited abduction and adduction of the right eye. The right palpebral fissure was vertically wider than the left, and there was slight downward displacement of the right lower lid. A moveable mass was palpable at the inferior lateral orbital rim. Orbital ultrasound showed a solid tumor mass.

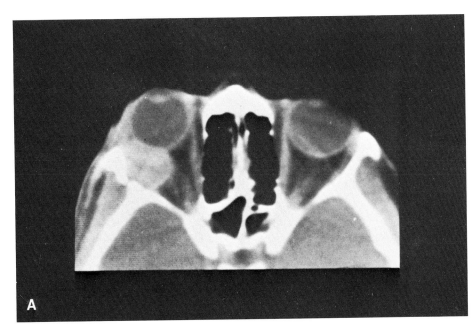

Figure A. The right globe is proptotic. A homogeneous contrast-enhancing mass is seen in the anterior lateral aspect of the right orbit. Some streaking artifacts from the adjacent bone cross through the tumor. The mass has smooth, well-defined margins. The deformity of the lateral wall of the orbit is related to the previous surgery. The mass appears to be both extraconal and intraconal.

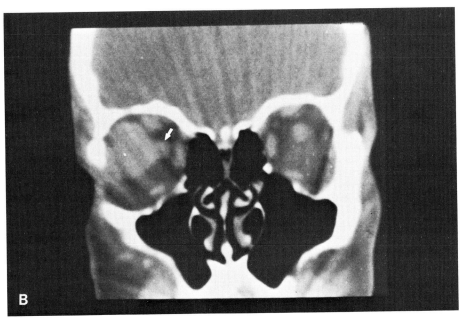

Figure B. Coronal scan. The optic nerve (arrow) is displaced medially by the tumor.

Surgical Findings: A hemangiopericytoma was found in the region of the lacrimal fossa. It had infiltrated the muscle cone and could not be completely removed.

CASE 8. Rhabdomyosarcoma

A 13-month-old male with a bulging left eye for one week. One month ago, he was treated with antibiotics for a presumed periorbital cellulitis.

Clinical Examination: Left proptosis with increased orbital resistance. There was minimal movement of the left eye, and nystagmus was noted on left lateral gaze. There was epibulbar injection and elevation of the retina medially.

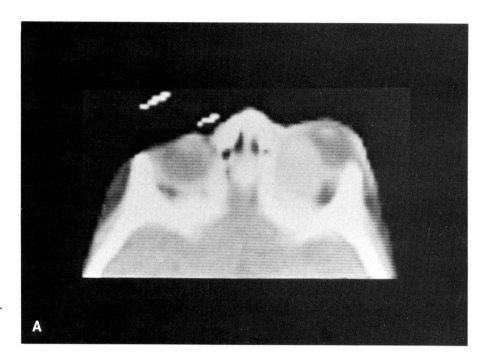

Figure A. CT scan shows a high-absorption, soft-tissue mass in the medial left orbit. The mass has smooth margins and a homogeneous appearance. The globe is displaced anteriorly and laterally.

Surgical Findings: An orbital exploration revealed an embryonal rhabdomyosarcoma. It could only be partially removed because it had completely infiltrated the medial rectus muscle.

CASE 9. Rhabdomyosarcoma
This young patient presented with right proptosis of a few weeks duration. Clinical examination revealed a soft-tissue mass in the medial aspect of the right orbit.

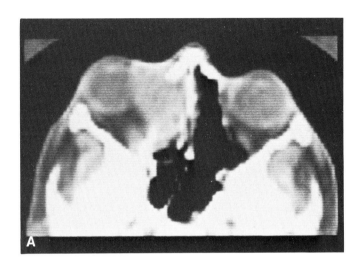

Figure A. The mass in the medial right orbit has destroyed the lamina papyracea and entered the adjacent ethmoid. The anterior and middle ethmoid cells are opacified. The mass is of slightly high absorption and relatively homogeneous. The globe is displaced anteriorly and laterally.

Follow-up: Biopsy revealed rhabdomyosarcoma, which was treated with radiation therapy. A follow-up scan was obtained a few months later.

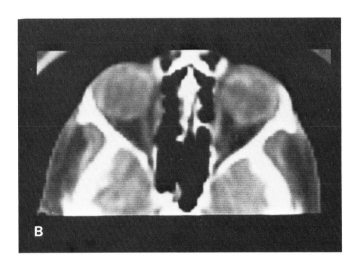

Figure B. Follow-up scan shows essentially complete resolution of the soft-tissue mass. The medial wall of the orbit and the globe are in normal position. The orbit and adjacent ethmoid sinus have a remarkably normal appearance.

CASE 10. Rhabdomyosarcoma

This is a 17-year-old male who had a 3-month history of a painful, red, watery right eye. The past two months he noticed increased swelling and bulging of the eye, blurred vision, diplopia, and nasal congestion. He was initially thought to have an orbital cellulitis and he was treated with IV antibiotics for seven days without improvement.

Clinical Findings: Marked proptosis with very limited extraocular movements of the right eye. A firm mass was palpable medial to the globe. Visual acuity was 20/40 OD and 20/20 OS. A 1.5 cm anterior cervical node was palpable on the right side.

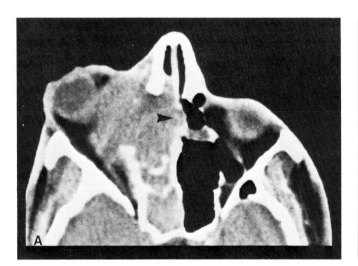

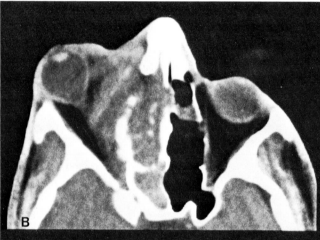

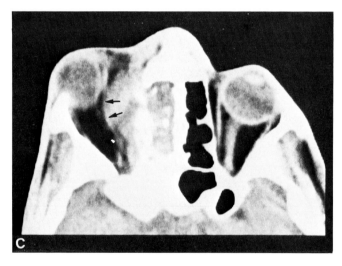

Figures A–C. Axial scans show a large soft-tissue mass involving the right ethmoid, nasal cavity, and medial orbit. The lamina papyracea and ethmoid septa are destroyed. The tumor has also eroded the perpendicular plate of the ethmoid (arrowhead) to enter the left nasal cavity. Superiorly (C) the structure bowed medially by the tumor is either the medial rectus or the superior oblique muscle (arrows). More inferiorly, the tumor certainly invades the muscle cone and appears to extend into the orbital apex. The right globe is displaced anteriorly and inferiorly.

Surgical Findings: A biopsy of polypoid tissue in his nose revealed a poorly differentiated tumor. This was followed by an ethmoidectomy and removal of the intranasal tumor with orbital decompression. Pathologic examination revealed an alveolar cell rhabdomyosarcoma. Patient then received both radiotherapy and chemotherapy.

CASE 11. Teratoma

A six-week-old male with congenital exophthalmos of the right eye.
Clinical Findings: Right proptosis. Absent light reflex and corneal reflex with
no eye movements. The left eye was normal. Angiography revealed a large
avascular mass in the right middle fossa extending posteriorly and associated with occlusion of the right internal carotid artery.

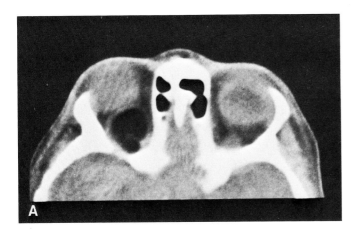

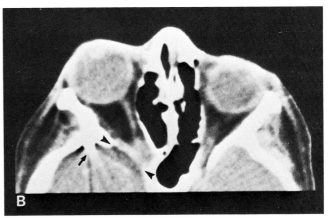

Figure A. A discrete mass is seen in the retrobulbar region of the right orbit. The mass has a smooth, well-defined rim and a low-density cystic center.

Figure B. The globe is proptotic, and the optic nerve is bowed medially. The superior orbital fissure (arrowheads) is markedly widened. The surgical clip (arrow) is related to a recent intracranial operation.

Surgical Findings: At the first operation a large, well-differentiated teratoma was found in the floor of the right
middle fossa. Approximately 1.5 mL of mucoid material was aspirated from the mass, indicating that it was partially
cystic. The mass extended posteriorly onto the tentorium. The tumor was not adherent to the brain, but because of
its large size it was only partially removed at the first operation. A repeat craniotomy was done one week later,
and the intracranial tumor was completely removed. Tumor was noted entering the orbit through a greatly expanded superior orbital fissure. The orbital component came out with a small amount of traction, and there was no
obvious attachment within the orbit.
Final Diagnosis: Benign teratoma.

CASE 12. Lymphoma

For the past 8 months this 77-year-old female had noticed left frontal headaches, gradually increasing proptosis, and decreasing vision in the left eye. *Clinical Findings:* A firm mass was palpable in the medial left orbit, associated with exotropia and corneal exposure. Orbital ultrasound revealed a solid retrobulbar mass that did not appear to invade the globe.

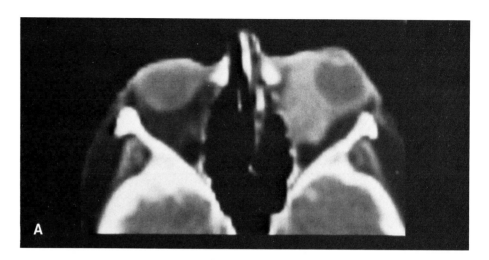

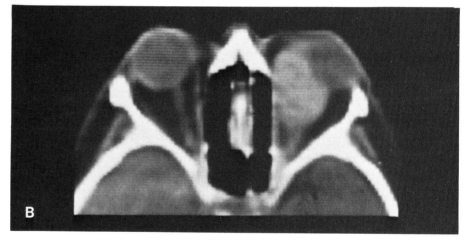

Figures A and B. Contrast scans demonstrate a contrast-enhancing mass in the medial left orbit that displaces the globe anteriorly and laterally. The mass is immediately adjacent to the globe and appears to involve both the extraconal and intraconal spaces. The margins are slightly lobulated but well demarcated by the orbital fat. No bone destruction is evident.

Diagnosis: A biopsy disclosed malignant lymphoma, lymphocytic type and poorly differentiated. The tumor responded to 4040 rad of radiation therapy, with a decrease of the proptosis and improvement of vision in the left eye.

CASE 13. Lymphoma
An 87-year-old female with marked right proptosis. Sixteen years ago an orbital biopsy was diagnosed as pseudotumor. She developed recently skin nodules on the arms and abdomen.

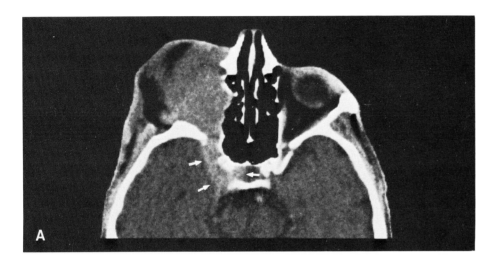

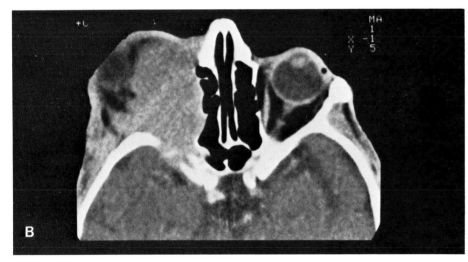

Figures A and B. Contrast scans show a large, homogeneous soft-tissue mass filling the right orbit. The margins are irregular in places, but the lamina papyracea is bowed medially, suggesting that the mass has been present for some time. The mass has eroded the superior orbital fissure and entered the intracranial cavity to involve the paracavernous and sella regions (arrows). The globe is displaced markedly anteriorly beyond the field of the scanner. The lateral orbital wall was previously removed.

Diagnosis: A biopsy of one of the skin nodules revealed lymphoma. The orbital lesion responded dramatically to 2000 rad of radiation therapy. The proptosis resolved completely following treatment.

CASE 14. Lymphoma

This is a 77-year-old female with a protruding left eye for the past 2 years. The proptosis increased in the past few months, and she developed an aching forehead pain.

Clinical Findings: Visual acuity, 20/25 OD and 20/30 OS. Fields were full. Exophthalmos of 6 mm was present on the left. She had increased orbital resistance, but ocular motility was normal. Orbital ultrasound revealed an ill-defined mass along the lateral wall of the left orbit.

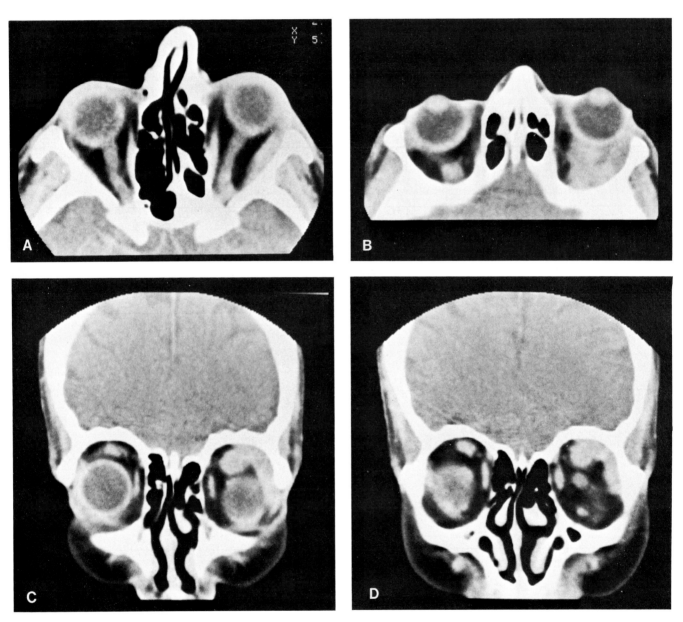

Figures A–D. CT scans show a soft-tissue mass in the superior lateral aspect of the left orbit, causing slight proptosis. The mass appears to be predominantly extraconal, but there is infiltration of the lateral and superior rectus muscles. The optic nerve is not involved. The margins of the mass are slightly irregular and ill-defined in some areas. The adjacent bone is not involved.

Follow-up: A Kronlein lateral orbitotomy was performed, and an extensive infiltrative tumor was found. Pathologic examination revealed a lymphoma of mixed type. Bone marrow biopsy, lymphangiogram, and serum immunoelectrophoresis showed no evidence of systemic disease. The tumor was treated with radiation therapy, and follow-up scans were obtained a few months later.

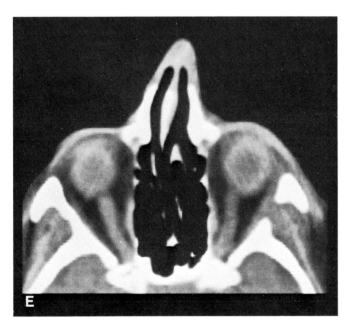
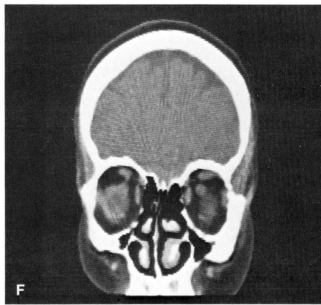

Figures E and F. CT scans show dramatic resolution of the orbital mass. There is some residual thickening of the soft tissues along the lateral wall of the left orbit. The bone defect is related to the lateral orbitotomy.

CASE 15. Lymphoma
This 78-year-old female noted swelling of her left eyelid about two months ago.
Clinical Findings: The left eye was protruding and displaced laterally. A 3 × 2-cm mass was palpable extending from the medial canthus of the left eye to the bridge of the nose.

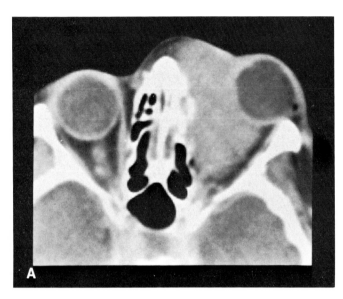

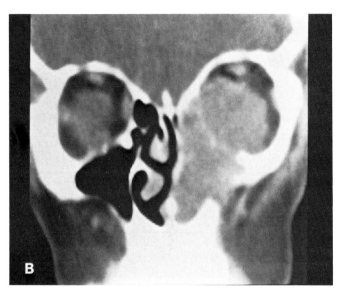

Figure A. Axial CT scan demonstrates a large soft-tissue mass in the medial left orbit. The mass involves the soft tissues anteriorly and has extended posteriorly in the retrobulbar region to approach the orbital apex. It involves both the extraconal and intraconal spaces. The mass is homogeneous, and it has an infiltrative appearance. The globe is slightly deformed and misplaced anteriorly and to the left.

Figure B. A coronal scan clearly shows the extent of the orbital involvement. There is erosion of the medial wall and floor of the orbit, with extension of the soft-tissue mass into the left ethmoid and maxillary sinuses and the left nasal cavity. Also noted is erosion in the lateral wall of the antrum. On this section the cribriform plate remains intact.

Follow-up: A biopsy revealed histiocytic lymphoma, which was treated with radiation therapy. No systemic involvement was evident at the time of presentation.

CASE 16. Lymphoma

This is a 52-year-old female with swelling of the right lower lid and increased tearing of the right eye for about 3 years. In the past few months she noticed displacement of the right eye and diplopia.

Clinical Findings: Slight exophthalmos and upward displacement of the right eye. A firm mass was palpable near the right medial canthus. Visual acuity was 20/25 OD and 20/20 OS. Visual fields were normal. Ultrasound showed a tubular mass lying along the medial wall of the right orbit. A dacryocysto-gram revealed obstruction of the nasal lacrimal duct at the level of the nasal lacrimal sac.

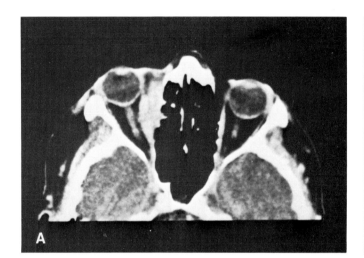 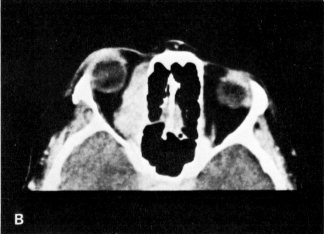

Figures A and B. Axial scans show a relatively homogeneous soft-tissue mass in the medial right orbit. It is extraconal but does infiltrate the medial rectus muscle and extends into the orbital apex. The margins are fairly well defined. The globe is displaced laterally and anteriorly. The adjacent ethmoid sinuses are normally aerated.

Follow-up: A biopsy revealed a histiocytic lymphoma, which was treated with radiation therapy.

CASE 17. Lymphoma

A 73-year-old male with a 10-month history of mild visual blurring and horizontal diplopia in the right lateral gaze.

Clinical Findings: A large irregular mass was palpable in the right lower lid and lateral aspect of the orbit. There was decreased orbital resilience and 4 mm of exophthalmos. Palpable lymph nodes were present in the neck and both axillae.

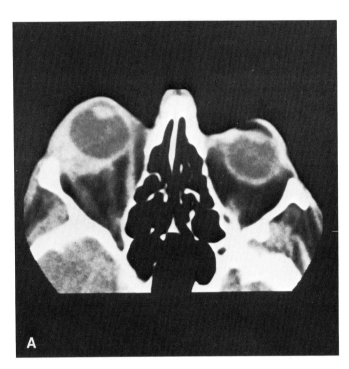 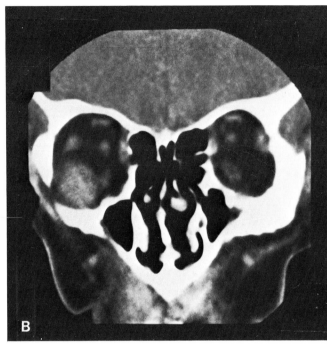

Figures A and B. Axial and coronal scans demonstrate a soft-tissue mass in the lateral and inferior aspects of the anterior right orbit. The mass has irregular margins and has a homogeneous appearance. The mass is present on both sides of the orbital septum and infiltrates the soft-tissue structures in the retrobulbar region, extending medially to reach the optic nerve. The globe is proptotic and displaced medially.

Follow-up: A biopsy of the mass revealed malignant lymphocytic lymphoma, well differentiated. A bone marrow biopsy was negative; however, because of the palpable lymph nodes, the patient was treated with chemotherapy.

CASE 18. Lymphoma

This 69-year-old male was admitted with a seven-month history of tearing and irritation of the right eye.

Clinical Findings: A mass was palpable in the medial inferior aspect of the right orbit without evidence of tenderness or erythema. Orbital ultrasound showed an irregular solid mass measuring 24 × 15 mm that did not extend posteriorly to the equator of the globe.

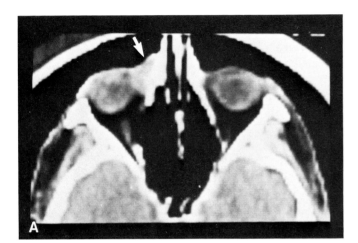 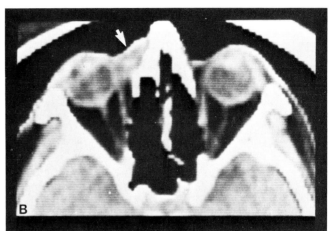

Figures A and B. Axial scans show a soft-tissue mass (arrow) anterior to the orbital septum in the medial right orbit. The globe is displaced laterally. The muscle cone does not appear to be invaded.

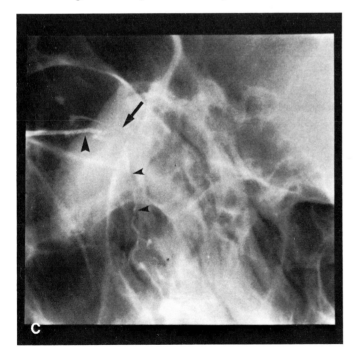

Figure C. An oblique view of a dacryocystogram. The cannula is inserted in the inferior canaliculus (large arrowhead). There is a high-grade obstruction of the lacrimal sac (arrow), with only a small amount of contrast material entering the nasal lacrimal duct (small arrowheads).

Follow-up: At surgery, a 15 × 15-mm invasive tumor was found originating from the lacrimal sac. Pathology revealed a malignant lymphoma of a mixed cell type. The patient was treated with 4000 rad of radiation therapy.

CASE 19. Lymphoma

This 88-year-old male had a 3- to 4-year history of left ptosis and progressive exophthalmos. His vision had been poor bilaterally for many years.

Clinical Findings: Left exophthalmos. There was also edema and ptosis of the left upper lid. Ultrasound confirmed a tumor in the muscle cone.

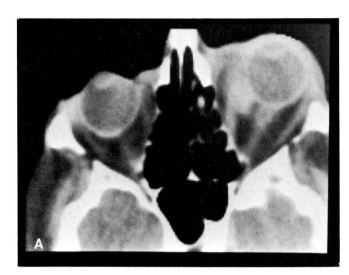 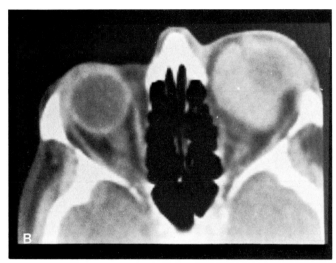

Figures A and B. CT scans show a homogeneous fairly well defined mass in the retrobulbar region of the left orbit. It is primarily intraconal but does extend anteriorly around the medial side of the globe. The globe is proptotic but is not invaded by the tumor. The mass is positioned superior to the optic nerve.

Surgical Findings: A left orbital exploration was done with partial excision of the tumor. Pathologic examination revealed lymphocytic lymphoma, well differentiated.

CASE 20. Schwannoma
This is a nine-year-old female with increasing proptosis over the past year.
She had two orbital explorations during that time.
Clinical Findings: At this time she had 5 mm of exophthalmos on the right.
There was limited adduction and abduction of the right eye. A prominent
subconjunctival vessel was noted at the right lateral canthal area.

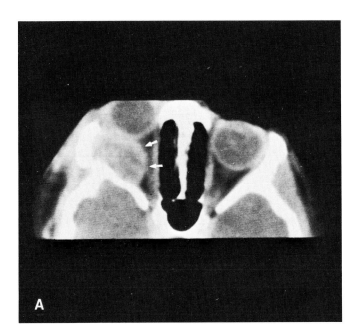
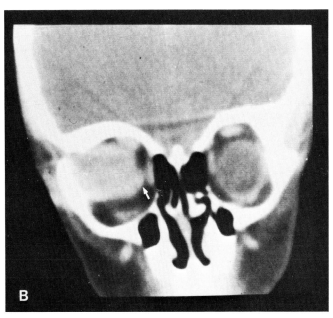

Figures A and B. The patient has had a previous lateral orbitotomy. Axial and coronal scans show a heterogeneous soft-tissue mass in the lateral aspect of the right orbit. The margins are well defined, and the mass involves
both the extraconal and intraconal compartments. The globe is displaced anteriorly and medially. The optic nerve
is not clearly defined but is identified medial to the mass (arrows).

Surgical Findings: Orbital exploration revealed a 30 × 25 × 20-mm schwannoma, which was completely excised.
The surgery included a curettage of the anterior portions of the frontal bone and superior lateral orbital rim.

CASE 21. Schwannoma
This is a 44-year-old female with proptosis OD for 5 years and poor vision in the right eye for 10 years. Recently she noted increasing proptosis and decreasing visual acuity. Orbital ultrasound revealed a large solid intraconal tumor.

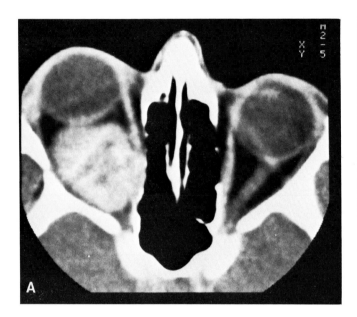

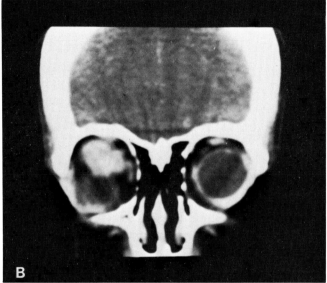

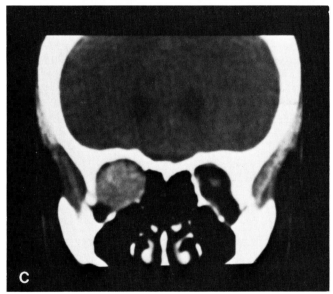

Figures A–C. Axial and coronal scans show a large high-absorption mass within the intraconal compartment of the right orbit. The margins are smooth and well defined. The right orbit is enlarged, with medial bowing of the lamina papyracea. The lateral and medial rectus muscles are compressed against the orbital walls by the mass and the globe is proptotic.

Surgical Findings: An orbital exploration revealed a large intraconal tumor, which could only be partially resected because it was adherent to the optic nerve. Pathologic examination showed a schwannoma.

CASE 22. Neurofibrosarcoma

This is a 55-year-old male with an 18-year history of a tumor in the right orbit. The patient had multiple surgeries in the past. Recently, the mass has been growing more rapidly.

Clinical Findings: Proptosis OD. The extraocular movements (EOMs) were nearly absent, and there was no vision in the right eye. No other cranial nerve deficits were noted.

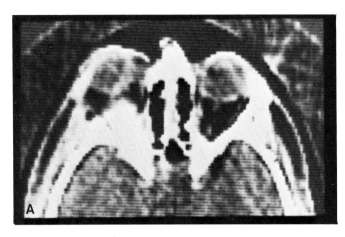

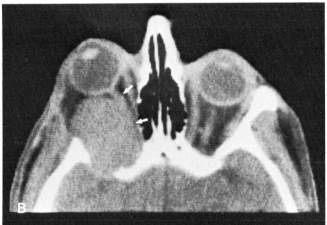

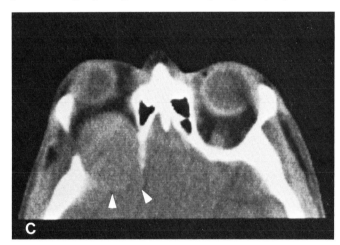

Figure A. A scan done 2½ years earlier showed a contrast-enhancing mass in the right orbital apex. The margins are slightly irregular and the right globe proptotic.

Figures B and C. Axial scans on the present admission demonstrate a large homogeneous mass in the posterior lateral aspect of the right orbit. The optic nerve (arrows) is stretched and displaced medially and the globe is proptotic. The margins are smooth and well defined. The mass has eroded the posterior wall of the orbit and bulges into the intracranial cavity (arrowheads). The patient has had a previous lateral orbitotomy.

Follow-up. The mass was resected through a subfrontal craniotomy. Pathologic examination revealed a neurofibroma with atypia suggestive of neurofibrosarcoma.

CASE 23. Dermoid Cyst

Patient with a several-year history of a mass in the left orbit. A soft-tissue mass was palpable in the anterior lateral aspect of the left orbit. The mass was slightly fluctuant and orbital resistance was normal. Extraocular movements and vision were also normal.

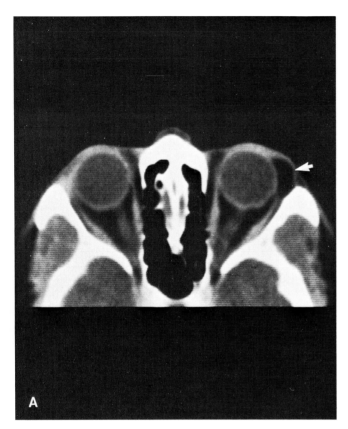 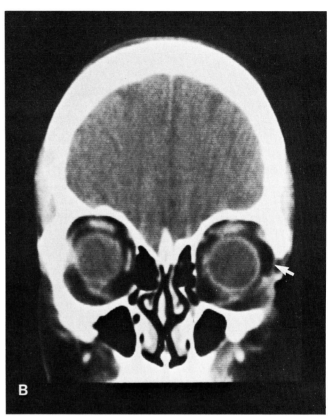

Figures A and B. Axial and coronal CT scans demonstrate a cystic mass (arrows) in the anterior lateral aspect of the left orbit. The mass is extraconal and anterior to the orbital septum. It has a smooth, thin rim and a low-absorption center. The retrobulbar structures are normal.

Follow-up: At surgery, a dermoid cyst was found and completely removed.

CASE 24. Dermoid Cyst
Patient with a 15-year history of an asymptomatic mass in the right orbit.

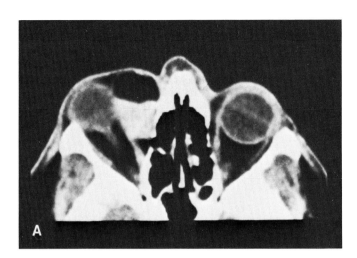

Figure A. There is a large mass in the medial extraconal space of the right orbit. The globe and the medial rectus muscle are displaced laterally, and the right orbit is enlarged. The anterior portion of the mass appears to be cystic and had Hounsfield numbers in the range of −100. The mass also contains high-density material that seems to be layering in the posterior portion of the mass. The mass is smoothly marginated and well defined.

Diagnosis: Dermoid cyst. Dermoid cysts often contain epithelial debris that can sediment into the dependent portion of the cyst.

CASE 25. Dermoid Cyst

A 43-year-old male with a prominent right eye for several years. This has particularly increased during the past 12 months. He had no pain, previous trauma, or thyroid disorder.

Clinical Findings: A mass was palpable in the superior aspect of the right orbit. There was limited elevation and abduction of the right eye. Orbital ultrasound showed a relatively homogeneous mass with few internal echoes.

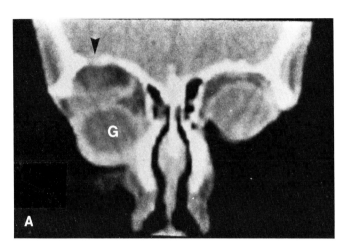 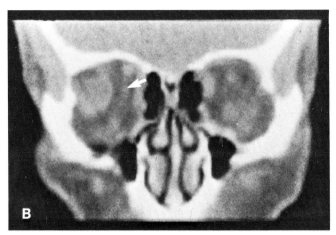

Figures A and B. Coronal scans demonstrate a mass in the superior aspect of the right orbit. The globe (G) is displaced markedly inferiorly. The mass has slightly irregular margins and a low-absorption center. There is deformity and focal erosion (arrowhead) of the adjacent orbital roof. The optic nerve (arrow) is displaced medially.*

Follow-up: With a lateral orbitotomy, the cystic tumor was completely removed. Pathologic examination revealed a dermoid cyst.

Reprinted from Hesselink JR, Davis KR, Dallow RL, et al: Computed tomography of masses in the lacrimal gland region. Radiology 131:146, 1979, with permission.

CASE 26. Dermoid Cyst
A 45-year-old patient with a mass in the right orbit for several years.

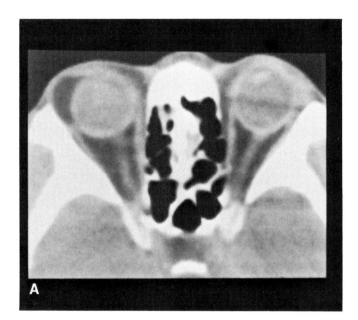 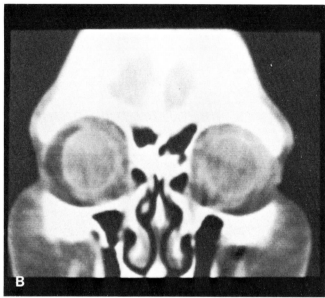

Figures A and B. Axial and coronal scans demonstrate a cystic mass in the anterior lateral aspect of the right orbit. The mass is extraconal and predominantly anterior to the orbital septum. It has well-defined margins and a low-absorption center. The globe is displaced slightly medially. The retrobulbar structures are normal.

Follow-up: Because of the minor symptoms, the patient declined surgery at this time. The CT findings are characteristic for a dermoid cyst.

CASE 27. Dermoid Cyst

A 24-year-old male with a mass in the left orbit for many years. The lesion has slowly enlarged over the past few years.

Clinical Findings: A soft-tissue mass was palpable in the superior lateral aspect of the left orbit. Slight hypotropia was present. Vision was normal. Orbital ultrasound showed a cystic lesion of the left orbit.

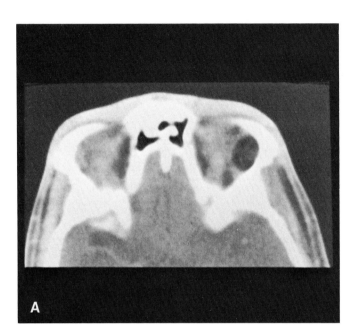 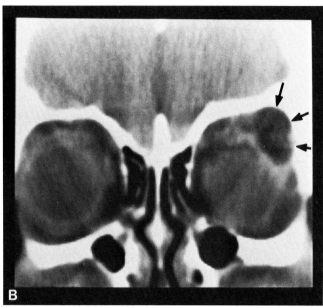

Figures A and B. Axial and coronal scans demonstrate a cystic mass in the left orbit. The mass is positioned anteriorly, lateral and superior to the globe. The mass has a cystic low-density center. The margins of the mass are somewhat ill defined, and soft-tissue density is present adjacent to the mass. There is erosion of the superior lateral aspect of the bony orbit (arrows).

Follow-up: At surgery, a cystic tumor was found and was completely excised. Pathologic examination revealed a dermoid cyst with secondary dacryoadenitis and inflammation of the adjacent orbital connective tissues.

CASE 28. Pleomorphic Adenoma of Lacrimal Gland
This 28-year-old female had noticed increased prominence of the right eye over the past 3 to 4 years. This was associated with a dull ache in the superior aspect of the right orbit, blurred vision, and intermittent diplopia. Physical examination revealed 6 mm of exophthalmos and increased orbital resistance; the right globe was displaced inferiorly. A firm, nontender mass was palpable in the upper temporal quadrant. Vision was 20/50 OD and 20/20 OS. Orbital ultrasound demonstrated a large mass with internal echoes consistent with a solid tumor.

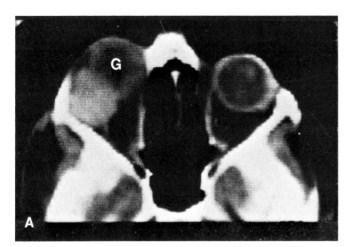 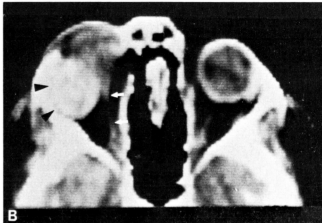

Figures A and B. Axial scans demonstrate a contrast-enhancing mass in the anterior lateral aspect of the right orbit. The mass is slightly heterogeneous and the margins are well defined. The globe (G) is displaced anteriorly, medially, and inferiorly. The optic nerve (arrows) is stretched and displaced medially. The mass is predominantly extraconal; however, involvement of the muscle cone cannot be excluded on these scans. Also noted is some erosion of the lateral orbital wall (arrowheads).

Surgical Findings: The tumor was excised via a lateral Kronlein approach. The mass had an intact capsule, and pathologic examination revealed a pleomorphic adenoma of the lacrimal gland.

CASE 29. Pleomorphic Adenoma of Lacrimal Gland

The chief complaint of this 70-year-old female was progressive painless exophthalmos of the left eye over 8 years. On physical examination, there was proptosis and increased orbital resistance. Also noted was ptosis, and the globe was displaced downward and medially. An irregular, firm, and fixed mass was palpable in the upper temporal quadrant. Orbital ultrasound revealed a large extraconal irregular mass with internal echoes consistent with solid tumor.

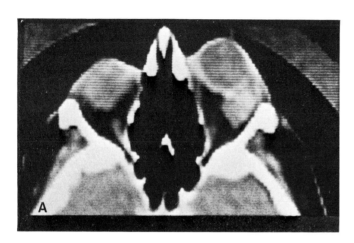

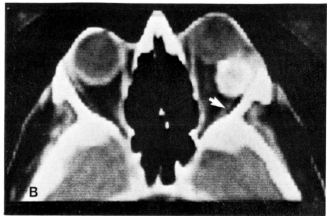

Figure A. A plain scan shows a soft-tissue mass in the anterior lateral aspect of the left orbit. The globe is displaced anteriorly and medially.

Figure B. A contrast scan shows moderate enhancement of the mass. The matrix of the mass is somewhat heterogeneous. It appears to involve both the extraconal and intraconal compartments because the lateral rectus muscle (arrow) is not displaced medially.

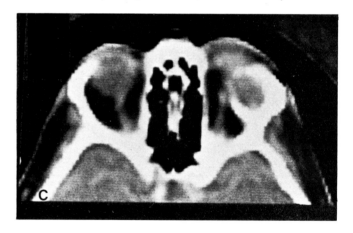

Figure C. A higher section shows bone surrounding the anterior and posterior aspects of the mass.

Surgical Findings: At surgery, the mass was firmly fixed and embedded in the lateral orbital wall. It had both solid and cystic components. The lateral rectus muscle was adherent to the inferior aspect of the mass, which explains why the lateral rectus muscle was not displaced medially by this extraconal mass. The final pathologic determination was pleomorphic adenoma of the lacrimal gland.

CASE 30. Adenocystic Carcinoma of Lacrimal Gland

This 27-year-old female had vague pain and progressive diplopia in the right orbit over the past few months. She also noted increased dryness of the right eye.

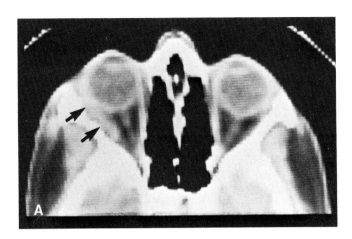

Figure A. There is an ill-defined soft-tissue mass lateral to the right globe (arrows) that extends posteriorly along the lateral rectus muscle. It does not appear to reach the orbital apex. There is irregularity of the adjacent bony orbit. The globe is slightly proptotic.

Surgical Findings: At surgery, an invasive tumor was found in the lacrimal fossa. It was adherent to the orbital plate of the frontal bone and the bone had a softened appearance. Pathologic examination revealed adenocystic carcinoma of the lacrimal gland with extension into the muscle and bone. Also noted on this specimen was penetration of vascular walls. Surgery was followed by 5400 rad of radiation therapy.

CASE 31. Adenocarcinoma of Lacrimal Gland

Over the past six months, this 47-year-old male had progressive right exophthalmos. Clinical examination revealed right lid lag, inflamed conjunctiva, limited upward gaze, and increased orbital resistance. A mass was also palpable at the lateral orbital rim. Vision was 20/40 OD and 20/20 OS. Orbital ultrasound showed thickened soft tissue along the lateral orbital wall, which was suspicious for invasive tumor.

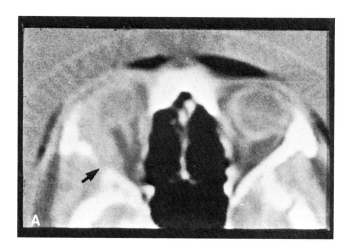

Figure A. CT scan shows an ill-defined soft-tissue mass in the lateral extraconal space of the right orbit. The globe is displaced medially. Also noted is erosion of the lateral wall of the orbit (arrow).*

Surgical Findings: Adenocarcinoma of the lacrimal gland was found at surgery. It invaded the right wall of the orbit and extended posteriorly to involve the greater wing of the sphenoid.

Reprinted from Hesselink JR, Davis KR, Dallow RL, et al: Computed tomography of masses in the lacrimal gland region. Radiology 131:145, 1979, with permission.

CASE 32. Benign Lymphoepithelial Lesion of Lacrimal Gland

A 47-year-old female with intermittent progressive swelling of the right upper
lid for 1 year.

Clinical Findings: A soft-tissue mass was palpable in the upper temporal
quadrant of the orbit at the rim. Also noted was ptosis of the right upper lid.
Orbital ultrasound showed a 1.5-cm mass in the right lacrimal gland.

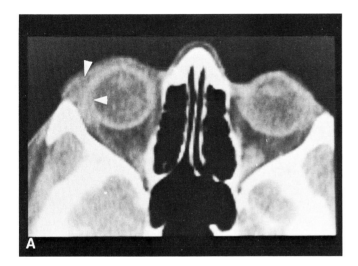
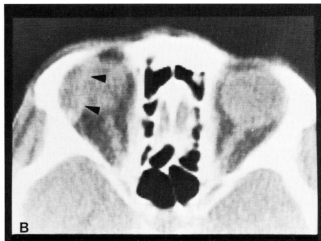

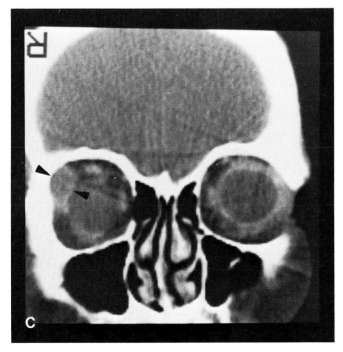

Figures A–C. Axial and coronal scans demonstrate a
focal soft-tissue mass (arrowheads) in the region of the
right lacrimal fossa. There are some areas of low density
within the mass. All of the margins are not clearly defined,
but it does not appear to invade the muscle cone. The
globe is displaced slightly medially and anteriorly.

Follow-up: With a lateral orbital approach, an oval mass of the lacrimal gland was removed from the right orbit.
Pathologic examination revealed lymphoid proliferation consistent with benign lymphoepithelial lesion of the lacrimal gland. Cystic areas were found within the mass. The patient remained asymptomatic, and there was no sign
of recurrence one year following the surgery.

CASE 33. Lymphocytic Infiltration of Lacrimal Gland

This 50-year-old female noted swelling and redness over the left upper and lower lids for about one month.

Clinical Findings: Vision was 20/20 OU. A mass was palpable beneath the left superior orbital rim. There was moderate limitation of upward gaze.

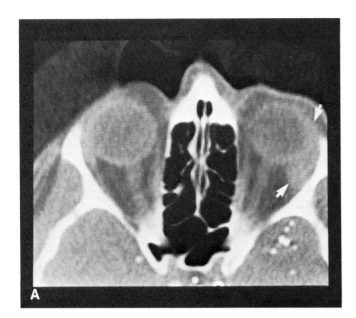 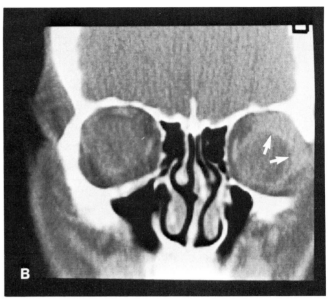

Figures A and B. Axial and coronal scans demonstrate a homogeneous soft-tissue mass (arrows) in the lacrimal region of the left orbit. The mass extends slightly posterior to the globe. The globe and optic nerve are displaced medially. On the coronal scan the mass is noted to extend around the globe from 11 o'clock to 4 o'clock. The edges of the mass are slightly irregular. No bone erosion is identified.

Follow-up: At surgery an 8 × 5-mm solid mass was found. It had a yellowish color, was avascular, and had a well-formed capsule. Pathologic examination revealed diffuse lymphocytic infiltration of the lacrimal gland, suggestive of Sjögren's syndrome.

CASE 34. Mikulicz Syndrome Involving the Lacrimal Glands
This 49-year-old female had marked bilateral exophthalmos associated with swelling of the submaxillary and parotid glands. Physical examination revealed 35 mm of exophthalmos bilaterally and enlargement of both lacrimal glands. Vision was 20/20 OU.

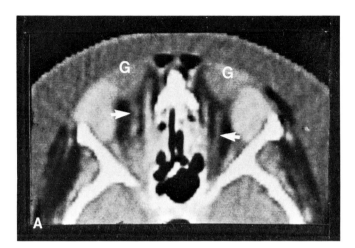 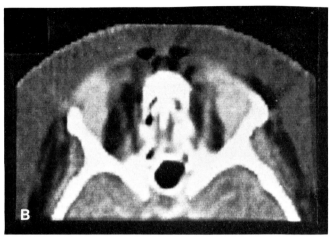

Figures A and B. There are sharply defined contrast-enhancing masses in both orbits. Both masses are in the lacrimal gland region, and they have a relatively homogeneous appearance. The globes (G) are markedly displaced anteriorly, and the optic nerves (arrows) are stretched.*

Surgical Findings: A biopsy of the right lacrimal gland was consistent with Mikulicz disease. A bilateral Kronlein orbital decompression was done.

Reprinted from Hesselink JR, Davis KR, Dallow RL, et al: Computed tomography of masses in the lacrimal gland region. Radiology 131:146, 1979, with permission.

CASE 35. Osteoma
This 74-year-old female had a 1-year history of slowly progressive diplopia on bilateral gaze associated with pain in the right eye. Clinical examination revealed 4 mm of proptosis OD and a mild decrease in extraocular movements. Vision and visual fields were normal.

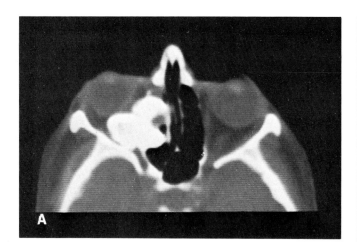 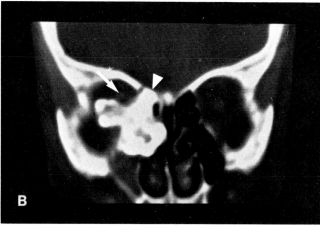

Figures A and B. Axial and coronal scans show a very dense mass along the medial wall of the right orbit. The mass occupies much of the ethmoid sinuses and bulges laterally into the orbit, causing slight proptosis. The margins are smooth and clearly defined. The optic nerve (arrow) is displaced superiorly and medially. The mass has also eroded the roof of the ethmoid (arrowhead) and also extended inferiorly to obstruct the osteum of the ipsilateral antrum.

Follow-up: At surgery, an osteoma was found, which was completely removed.

CASE 36. Osteoma

A mild but steady aching pain behind the right eye prompted this young male
to see a physician. Physical examination was entirely normal.

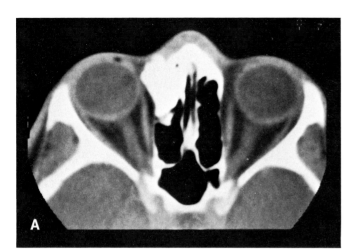 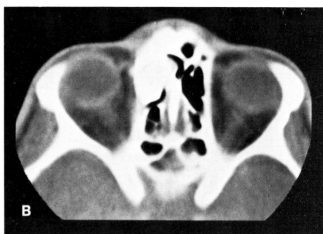

Figures A and B. There is a very dense mass in the anterior medial aspect of the right orbital wall. The mass fills the anterior ethmoid cells and bulges medially into the adjacent extraconal space of the orbit.

Follow-up: Because of the mild nature of the symptoms, the patient elected not to have surgery at this time. CT findings are characteristic of an osteoma.

CASE 37. Ewing's Sarcoma
This is a 66-year-old female with prominence of the left eye and left temporal region for several months. Visual acuity was 20/20 OU. The mass was very vascular on an arteriogram.

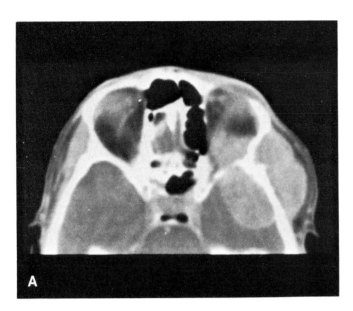 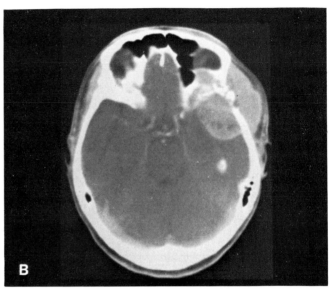

Figures A and B. Axial scans through the superior orbits demonstrate a large contrast-enhancing mass centered over the left greater sphenoid wing. Frank bone destruction is evident and soft-tissue mass bulges into the adjacent left orbit, temporal fossa, and middle cranial fossa. No calcification is evident within the mass, and it is relatively homogeneous except for a few areas of lower density posteriorly.

Follow-up: A left frontotemporal craniotomy and orbital decompression were performed. Pathologic examination disclosed a round-cell sarcoma. Differential included Ewing's sarcoma, clear-cell carcinoma of the tendon sheath, and rhabdomyosarcoma, although lymphoma and small-cell carcinoma also could not be excluded on the routine histologic examination. Electron microscopy was most consistent with Ewing's sarcoma.

CASE 38. Fibrous Dysplasia

This is a 20-year-old male with prominence of the left alveolar ridge, cheek, and forehead and elevation of the left globe. The patient had normal extra-ocular movements.

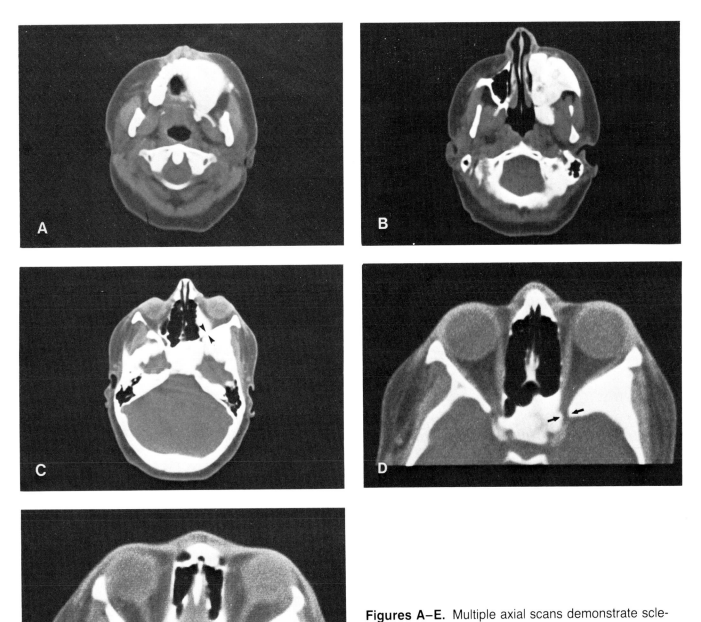

Figures A–E. Multiple axial scans demonstrate sclerotic hypertrophic bone involving the left superior alveolar ridge, maxilla, zygoma, base of sphenoid, and greater sphenoid wing. The left antrum is completely obliterated (Fig. B). Figure C shows considerable narrowing of the inferior orbital fissure (arrowheads). Compromise of the superior orbital fissure (arrows) is evident in Figure D.

Follow-up: The CT findings are characteristic of fibrous dysplasia. No surgery was recommended at this time.

CASE 39. Fibrous Dysplasia

Increased density of the right ethmoid was noted on skull films obtained for unrelated symptoms in this young male.

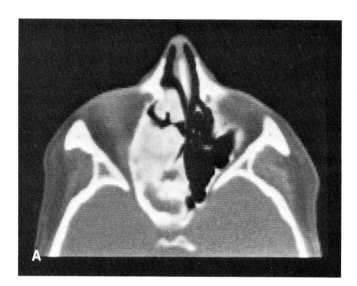 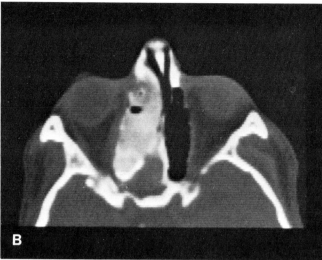

Figures A and B. There is a sclerotic process involving the right ethmoid and sphenoid sinuses. The sclerotic bone bulges into the medial right orbit and into the right nasal cavity.

Follow-up: No surgery was done. The radiographic and CT findings were characteristic of fibrous dysplasia.

CASE 40. Fibrous Dysplasia

This is a 46-year-old female with progressively decreasing vision in her right eye over the past few months.

Clinical Findings: Decreased visual acuity and absent color perception OD. Optic atrophy was also noted. The left eye was entirely normal.

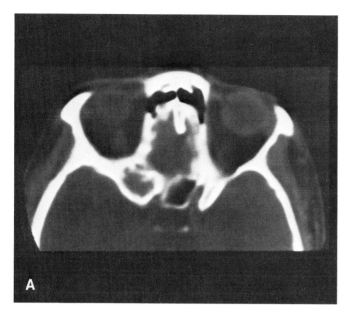

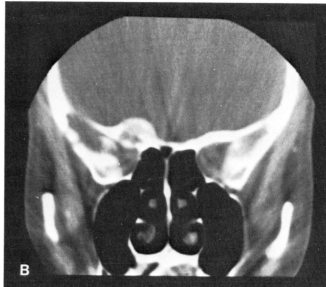

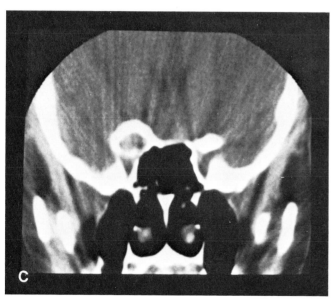

Figures A–C. Axial and coronal scans demonstrate an expansile sclerotic process involving the greater and lesser wings of the right sphenoid. The osseous mass obliterates the right optic canal and bulges into the orbital apex. No associated soft-tissue mass is identified.

Follow-up: No surgery was done. The CT findings are most consistent with fibrous dysplasia.

CASE 41. Cementifying Fibroma

This 24-year-old female first had surgery in Brazil in 1962 for an intracranial suprasellar lesion. After surgery, the vision in her left eye was reduced to counting fingers. In 1972, she developed right exophthalmos and infection of the frontal, ethmoid, and sphenoid sinuses. Via an external ethmoid approach, a mucocele of the sphenoethmoid region was removed. Presently she has bilateral proptosis, more marked on the right side and associated with increasing blurring of vision of the right eye.

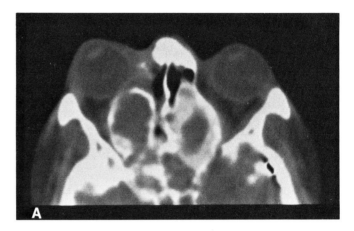

Figure A. Bilateral proptosis is evident. There is an expansile mass involving the sphenoid and both ethmoid sinuses. The mass bulges medially into both retrobulbar regions and certainly involves the region of the right optic canal, which would account for the decreasing vision. Recurrent mucocele formation cannot be excluded.

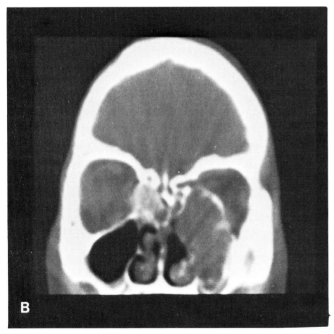

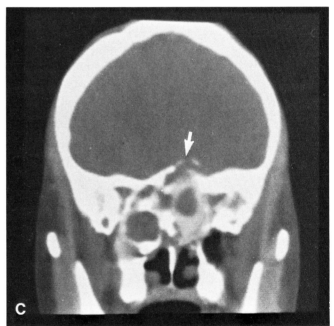

Figures B and C. On coronal scans, the expansile mass also involves the left antrum and nasal cavity. There is also erosion of the roof of the sphenoid on the left side with bulging of the mass into the anterior cranial fossa (arrow).

Follow-up: Surgical drainage of a recurrent mucopyocele was done. Pathologic examination revealed a cementifying fibroma, a variant of fibrous dysplasia.

CHAPTER FIVE

Secondary and Metastatic Tumors of the Orbit

In a series of 764 tumors seen at the Mayo Clinic, 45 percent, or nearly half, were secondary or extraorbital tumors with direct extension into the orbit.[1] Since the orbits are surrounded by the paranasal sinuses and intracranial cavity, they are vulnerable to spread of diseases from these neighboring areas. Lymphatic spread cannot occur because the orbit has no lymphatics, but tumors can infiltrate along perivascular and perineural spaces, as well as through orbital foramina. Metastatic disease to the eye and orbit also is not rare, accounting for 3 percent of patients with unilateral exophthalmos at the Columbia Eye Institute[2] and 7 percent of the orbital tumors in the Mayo Clinic's series.[1] Metastases spread via the bloodstream from primary site to some distant site.

SECONDARY TUMORS

Various pathways are available for orbital extension of extraorbital diseases. Thin bony walls separate the orbit from the surrounding paranasal sinuses. The orbit also communicates with other compartments of the face and intracranial cavity through multiple normal foramina. The method of entry into the orbit depends on the histology and location of the tumor.[3]

Sinuses *(Cases 1–5)*
In the early stages, neoplasms of the paranasal sinuses are clinically silent or may masquerade as a benign sinusitis. Too often the presence of a malignancy is heralded by symptoms related to spread beyond the sinuses. It is not unusual for a sinus tumor to present with proptosis. Other signs of orbital involvement include restriction of eye movement, congestion of the conjunctiva, and orbital pain.[4]

Since the sinuses are lined by epithelium, it is not unexpected that carcinomas represent 80 percent of all sinus malignancies. Of these, 90 percent are squamous cell carcinoma. Less common types include adenocarcinoma and adenocystic carcinoma. The other 20 percent of sinus malignancies are sarcomas and lymphomas.[5]

Eighty percent of sinus carcinomas occur in the maxillary sinus. They are more likely to involve the orbit if they arise in the roof of the antrum. These tumors are very aggressive and simply destroy the orbit to enter the inferior extraconal space. Although carcinoma of the ethmoid is less common (5 to 6 percent), it more readily involves the orbit through the thin lamina papyracea. In fact, if orbital involvement by sinus carcinoma is seen, it is equally likely to be of ethmoid as maxillary origin. Ethmoid carcinoma also involves the nasal cavity early, causing nasal obstruction and bloody discharge. Because of their unique position, tumors of the sphenoid sinus have quite different characteristics. They readily erode into the sella turcica and extend into the parasellar and suprasellar regions. Involvement of the orbital apex can lead to cranial nerve palsies and superior orbital fissure syndrome. If the optic pathways are infiltrated or compressed, vision may be impaired. Neoplasms of the frontal sinus are rare. When they occur, they can destroy the floor of the sinus to enter the orbit.[6]

Sinus malignancies are infiltrating lesions and appear on a CT scan as homogeneous mass lesions with irregular margins. They are of average absorption on plain scan and demonstrate mild contrast enhancement. Bone destruction is common and can be extensive. Once the tumor enters the orbit, proptosis soon develops. At first, only the extraconal space of the orbit may be involved, but these tumors rapidly progress to infiltrate other structures within the orbit. The CT scan is particularly helpful in assessing extension into the orbital apex and intracranial cavity.[7,8]

In the Mayo Clinic's series,[1] mucoceles of the paranasal sinuses were included as secondary tumors. Although mucoceles are benign, they certainly behave as mass lesions, slowly enlarging to expand and erode adjacent bony structures. The frontal and ethmoid sinuses are the most common sites for mucoceles, and orbital involvement is common. In fact, frontoethmoid mucoceles often present with proptosis or a mass in the superior medial quadrant of the orbit. Progressive compression of the orbital contents may lead to visual impairment and even optic atrophy due to excessive stretching of the optic nerve.[9]

The density of a mucocele on CT scan depends on whether it contains clear mucous or thick viscous material of a pyocele. The majority are of average density and appear homogeneous. In general, they do not enhance, but acutely infected mucopyoceles may show enhancement of the wall. The margins are smooth and well defined. Mucoceles tend to displace bony margins rather than destroy them, so they are often bound by a thin rim of bone. Occasionally, an aggressive mucocele will expand so rapidly that it does not allow for bone remodeling. Nevertheless, as these mucoceles expand into the orbit, they displace normal orbital structures, in contrast to the infiltrating nature of a neoplasm.[10]

Nose and Nasopharynx (Cases 6 and 7)

Squamous cell carcinoma is also the most common malignant tumor of the nose and nasopharynx. Lymphoepithelioma is a treacherous variant of squamous cell carcinoma that is prone to metastasize as well as infiltrate locally. These tumors often spread to the skull base and track along the nerves to enter the cranial cavity. Malignant melanoma also occurs in the nasal cavity.[6] Esthesioneuroblastoma arises in the nasal cavity and region of the cribriform plate. They are very vascular and aggressive tumors. Tumors of the nose and nasal cavity usually reach the orbit via the ethmoid and maxillary sinuses. A more direct route is through the nasolacrimal duct, which connects the orbit with the inferior meatus of the nose.[3]

Infratemporal Fossa and Pterygopalatine Fossa (Cases 8 and 9)

Tumors in these compartments have direct access to the orbit through the inferior orbital fissure. Angiofibromas commonly involve the pterygopalatine fossa and extend into the infratemporal fossa, displacing the posterior lateral wall of the antrum forward. Characteristically, they have well-defined margins and show moderate to marked homogeneous enhancement. Extension into the orbit may be associated with widening of the inferior orbital fissure. Angiofibromas are very hypervascular, and even without direct orbital involvement, the existence of collateral venous drainage through the orbit may result in orbital congestion and proptosis.[3,11]

Neurofibromas arising in the infratemporal fossa can also involve the orbit. They are benign and well-defined masses. They are usually high-absorption areas on plain scan and enhance moderately with contrast.[12]

Superficial Face

Any tumors of the superficial facial structures have direct access to the orbit anteriorly. A basal cell carcinoma, sarcoma, or lymphoma of the skin and subcutaneous tissue can enter the orbit via the anterior route. These tumors are invasive and have irregular, poorly defined margins on CT (see Chapter 8, Case 29).

Intracranial Cavity (Cases 10–14)

Meningioma is by far the most common intracranial tumor to involve the orbit. Sphenoid wing meningiomas characteristically produce exuberant hyperostosis on both the orbital and middle fossa sides of the sphenoid wing. The hyperostotic bone encroaches on the extraconal spaces of the orbit and results in exophthalmos. Occasionally, an aggressive meningioma will destroy the sphenoid wing and enter the orbit directly. An alternative route to involve the orbit is through the superior orbital fissure. This is a more frequent route for meningiomas of a lesser sphenoid wing, tuberculum sella, and parasellar region. Hyperostosis associated with these meningiomas can also compromise the optic foramen, leading to visual impairment and optic atrophy.

The CT features of meningioma include high density on plain scan, marked homogeneous contrast enhancement, and clearly defined smooth margins. The bone changes are quite obvious on the CT scan, and calcification may be found in these tumors. The CT scan is particularly helpful for detecting extension into the orbital apex and for assessing the effect of the hyperostosis on the orbital structures.[3]

Chiasmatic and hypothalamic gliomas readily track anteriorly along the optic nerve to enter the orbit through the optic foramen. These tumors are low grade, but their location makes them unresectable. They are usually isodense on plain scan and demonstrate moderate contrast enhancement.

The floor of the anterior cranial fossa has rather thick bone and provides a strong barrier to the advance of tumor, but occasionally a glioblastoma of the frontal lobe may erode the floor of the anterior cranial fossa and invade the orbit. Glioblastomas are of low density on plain scan and elicit moderate to marked contrast enhancement. Also, chordomas can be very destructive and extend anteriorly to reach the orbital apex.

ORBITAL METASTASES (Cases 15–23)

Metastases to the orbit can occur in the globe, retrobulbar soft tissues and bony orbit. In our series of 34 patients, equal numbers of metastases were found in these three locations.[13] In a large series of 227 cases of carcinoma metastatic to the orbit, Ferry and Font[14] found that 86 percent were in the globe and 12 percent in the rest of the orbit. The incidence of ocular metastases depends on how hard one looks for them, because most are asymptomatic and are not detected. Metastases to the optic nerve are rare, only three cases occurring in Ferry and Font's large series. Pulmonary metastases accompany orbital metastases in 80 to 85 percent of cases.

The vast majority of orbital metastases in adults are carcinomas, and by far the most common primary sites are the breast and lung. Gastrointestinal, genitourinary, and thyroid sites are also seen. Metastatic melanoma is more common than primary melanoma of the choroid.[14]

The more common sources of orbital metastases in children are neuroblastoma, Ewing's sarcoma, and Wilm's tumor. These are embryonal tumors comprised of primitive or blastomatous elements. In contrast to adults, these tumors seem to metastasize exclusively to the orbit rather than the globe. In Albert's pathologic study of 46 cases of neuroblastoma and Ewing's sarcoma metastatic to the orbit in children, there were no ocular metastases.[15]

Ocular metastases usually present with blurred vision and increasing scotomata due to retinal detachment. They are most common in the posterior choroid on the temporal side near the macula, where the short posterior arteries are larger and more numerous.[2] As the tumor grows, it infiltrates along the choroid, progressively detaching and lifting the retina. The sclera is a strong barrier to an invasive tumor, but tumor can extend posteriorly through the lamina cribosa to involve the optic nerve and retrobulbar structures.

Choroidal metastases are usually small and are best evaluated with fundoscopy and orbital ultrasound. The CT scan is often negative; however, the choroidal mass can occasionally be detected as a focal area of enhancement. CT is most helpful for evaluating extraocular extension.

Exophthalmos is the most common symptom of metastases to the retrobulbar soft tissues. Associated findings include pain, decreasing vision, periorbital edema, ophthalmoplegia, and diplopia.[14] The majority of retrobulbar metastases occur in the extraconal space, but larger lesions involve both the extraconal and intraconal compartments. The features of retrobulbar metastases are variable and usually are nonspecific for the histology of the tumor. Most are high-absorption areas on plain scan and exhibit slight contrast enhancement.

They are relatively homogeneous and appear as discrete masses with irregular margins. An infiltrating mass with enophthalmos is characteristic of scirrhous carcinoma of the breast.[13]

The greater wing of the sphenoid is the most common orbital site of bone metastases. When a metastasis extends beyond the cortical bone, it encroaches on both the lateral extraconal space of the orbit and the middle cranial fossa. The CT appearance may simulate an aggressive meningioma. The distinction usually is not difficult because metastases are more destructive, and meningiomas enhance more with contrast and are more vascular at angiography.[13]

REFERENCES

1. Henderson JW: Orbital Tumors. New York, Theime-Stratton, 1980, pp 15–74, 425–496
2. Reese AB: Metastatic tumors of the eye and adnexa. In Tumors of the Eye. New York, Harper & Row, 3rd ed, 1976, Chap 16
3. Hesselink JR, Weber AL: Pathways of orbital extension of extraorbital neoplasms. J Comput Assist Tomogr 6(3):593–597, 1982
4. Mohan H, Sen D, Gupta D: Orbital affection in nasal and paranasal neoplasms. Acta Ophthalmol 47:289–294, 1963
5. Conley JJ: Sinus tumors invading the orbit. Trans Am Acad Ophthalmol Otolaryngol 70:615–619, 1966
6. Batsakis J: Tumors of the Head and Neck. Baltimore, Williams & Wilkins, 1974, pp 177–199
7. Hesselink JR, New PFJ, Davis KR, et al: Computed tomography of the paranasal sinuses and face: Part II. Pathological anatomy. J Comput Assist Tomogr 5:568–576, 1978
8. Bilaniuk LT, Zimmerman RA: Computer-assisted tomography: Sinus lesions with orbital involvement. Head Neck Surg 2:293–301, 1980
9. Wolfowitz BL, Solomon A: Mucoceles of the frontal and ethmoid sinuses. J Laryngol Otol 86:79–82, 1972
10. Hesselink JR, Weber AL, New PFJ, et al: Evaluation of mucoceles of the paranasal sinuses with computed tomography. Radiology 133:397–400, 1979
11. Osborn AG: Radiology of the pterygoid plates and pterygopalatine fossa. AJR 132:389–394, 1979
12. Doubleday LC, Jing BS, Wallace S: Computed tomography of the infratemporal fossa. Radiology 138:619–624, 1981
13. Hesselink JR, Davis KR, Weber AL, Davis JM, Taveras JM: Radiological evaluation of orbital metastases with emphasis on computed tomography. Radiology 137:363–366, 1980
14. Ferry AP, Font RL: Carcinoma metastatic to the eye and orbit. I. A clinicopathological study of 227 cases. Arch Ophthalmol 92:276–286, 1974
15. Albert DM, Rubenstein RA, Scheie HG: Tumor metastasis to the eye. Part II. Clinical study in infants and children. Am J Ophthalmol 63:727–732, 1967

CASE 1. Squamous Cell Carcinoma of Maxillary Sinus

This is a 63-year-old female with a 2½-month history of submandibular adenopathy, left proptosis, and maxillary sinusitis. A left neck mass was clinically palpable.

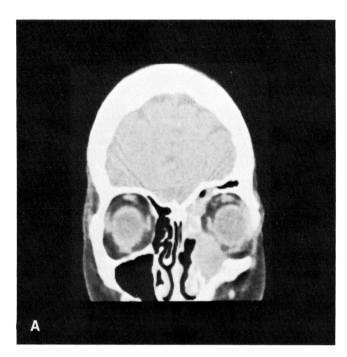 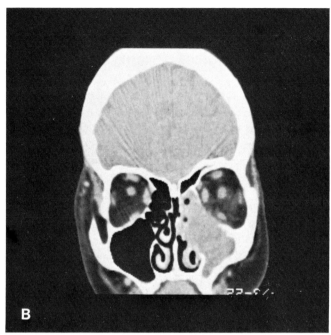

Figures A and B. Coronal scans demonstrate a soft-tissue mass in the left maxillary and ethmoid sinuses. The mass has destroyed the inferior and medial walls of the left orbit to involve the extraconal space. There is also erosion of the ethmoid septa and the ethmoidal maxillary plate, as well as of the medial wall of the antrum with extension of tumor into the nasal cavity.

Follow-up: The mass in the left nasal cavity was biopsied, which revealed squamous cell carcinoma.

CASE 2. Undifferentiated Carcinoma of Ethmoid

This 47-year-old female had right-sided headaches for about three months. The past 10 to 14 days she noted that the right eye was becoming more prominent.

Clinical Findings: There was moderate ptosis and increased orbital resistance on the right side. Cranial nerves were normal and the visual acuity was 20/20 OU with full visual fields.

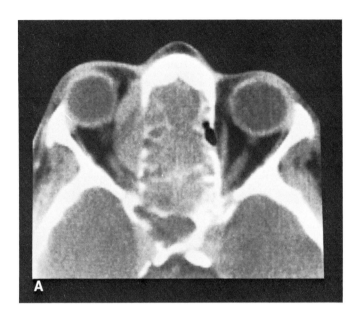   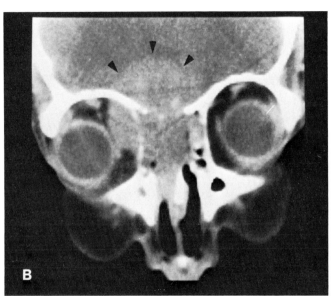

Figure A. Axial scan shows a soft-tissue mass involving both ethmoid sinuses. The mass has destroyed many of the ethmoid septa and the perpendicular plate and occupies both superior nasal cavities. There is erosion of the medial wall of the right orbit and soft-tissue mass bulges into the orbit.*

Figure B. On a coronal scan, the mass has destroyed the roof of the right ethmoid and the cribriform plates to extend into the intracranial cavity (arrowheads). The component in the right orbit displaces the globe laterally and inferiorly. Although the mass in the orbit has relatively well defined margins, the extent of bone destruction indicates an aggressive lesion.*

Follow-up: Surgery consisted of a right external ethmoidectomy and biopsy of the mass. An undifferentiated carcinoma was found, which was treated with radiation therapy.

*Reprinted from Hesselink JR, Weber AL: Pathways of orbital extension of extraorbital neoplasms. J Comput Assist Tomogr 6:595, 1982, with permission.

CASE 3. Mucocele

This is a 57-year-old male with increasing prominence of the left eye over the past five months.

Clinical Findings: Moderate exophthalmos OS. Vision was normal.

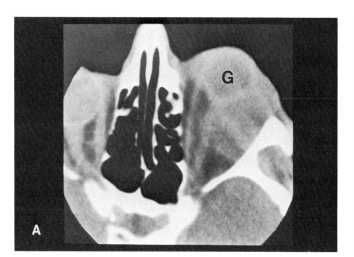

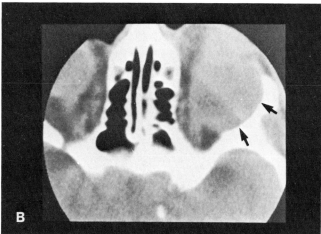

Figures A–C. Axial scans demonstrate a soft-tissue mass in the superior lateral aspect of the left orbit associated with an expansile process in the left frontal sinus. The mass appears to be relatively homogeneous despite some scan artifacts crossing the mass. The globe (G) is proptotic and optic nerve is stretched. The deformity of the lateral orbital wall (arrows) suggests a benign mass that has been present for some time. The expanding mass in the frontal sinus has eroded the posterior wall in areas (arrowheads).

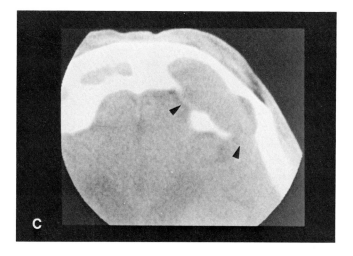

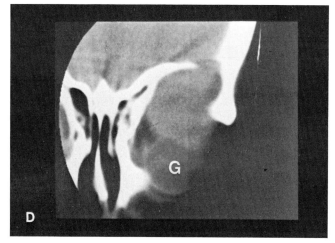

Figure D. A coronal scan clearly shows a mass in the left frontal sinus that has extended through the orbital roof. The margins of the mass are slightly irregular but well defined. The globe (G) is markedly displaced inferiorly.

Surgical Findings: At surgery, a frontal sinus mucocele that extended inferiorly into the orbit was found. Following drainage and curettage of the frontal sinus, the patient was discharged on tetracycline.

CASE 4. Mucocele

Progressive proptosis of the right eye was noted in this 60-year-old male over the past year. This was associated with intermittent right frontal headaches and increased tearing of the right eye.

Clinical Findings: A rubbery mass was palpable in the medial right orbit, which displaced the globe down and out. Vision was normal, but the ocular motility was decreased.

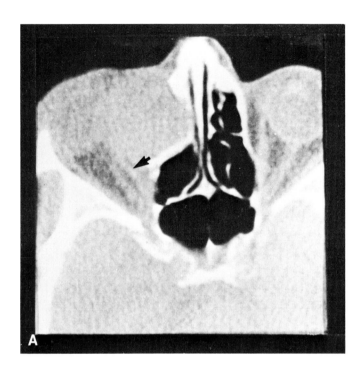
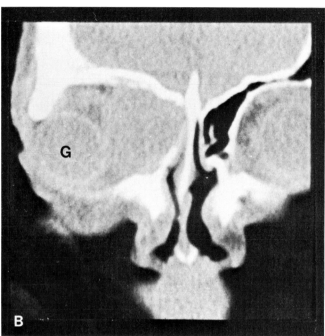

Figures A and B. Axial and coronal scans show a soft-tissue mass in the anterior right ethmoid sinuses that has destroyed the medial wall of the orbit and bulges into the orbit. The medial rectus muscle (arrow) is displaced laterally, suggesting the extraconal position of the mass. The globe (G) is displaced anteriorly, laterally, and inferiorly. The roof of the right ethmoid is displaced superiorly, suggesting the benign nature of the mass.

Follow-up: A frontal ethmoid mucocele was found; it was treated with an osteoplastic frontal obliteration.
Comment: Occasionally a rapidly expanding mucocele as in this case will destroy bone and simulate a neoplasm.

CASE 5. Mucocele

This 26-year-old female had a six-day history of progressive right orbital pain associated with mild edema of the right upper lid. No orbital mass was palpable.

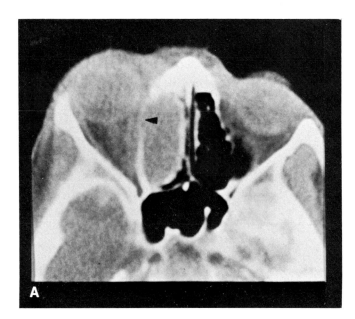 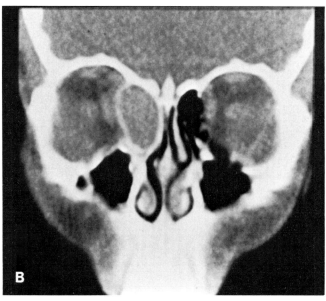

Figures A and B. Axial and coronal scans show a homogeneous expansile mass of the right ethmoid. The lamina papyracea is pushed and bowed laterally into the adjacent orbit. A focal area of erosion is noted anteriorly (arrowhead).*

Follow-up: A right external ethmoidectomy was performed. An ethmoid mucopyocele was found and, dehiscence of the lamina papyracea was noted in multiple areas. The contents of the mucocele were thick and purulent and *Staphylococcus aureus* grew on culture.

Figure A reprinted from Hesselink JR, Weber AL, New, PFJ, et al: Evaluation of mucoceles of the paranasal sinuses with computed tomography. Radiology 133:398, 1979, with permission.

CASE 6. Nasal Polyposis with Ethmoid Mucocele
A 37-year-old male with a history of allergic rhinitis and sinusitis recently noted increasing prominence of the right eye.

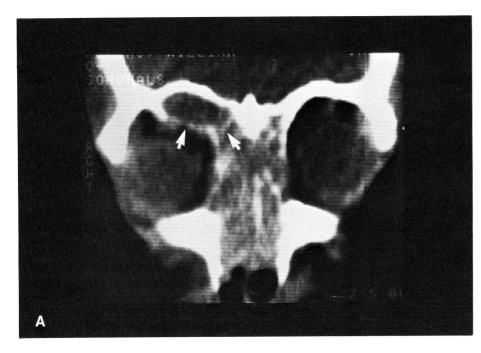

Figure A. On a coronal scan there is opacification of both nasal cavities and ethmoid sinuses. This is associated with erosion of the ethmoid septa and the perpendicular plate. A discrete expansile mass (arrows) in the right supraorbital ethmoid cell bulges into the superior medial aspect of the right orbit and displaces the globe inferiorly. Also noted is erosion of the superior medial wall of the orbit.*

Surgical Findings: At surgery, polypoid tissue filled the nasal cavities and ethmoid sinuses. A mucocele was found in the supraorbital cell of the right ethmoid.

*Reprinted from Hesselink JR, Weber AL, New PFJ, et al: Evaluation of mucoceles of the paranasal sinuses with computed tomography. Radiology 133:399, 1979, with permission.

CASE 7. Melanoma of the Nasal Cavity

This 62-year-old male presented because of persistent tearing in the right eye. On physical examination a large mass was noted in the inferior meatus of the right nasal cavity.

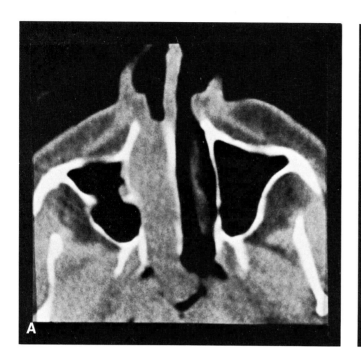

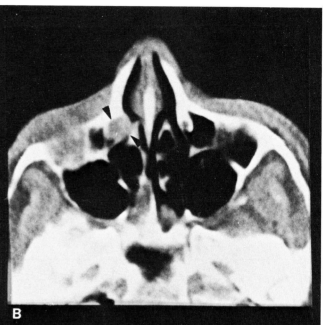

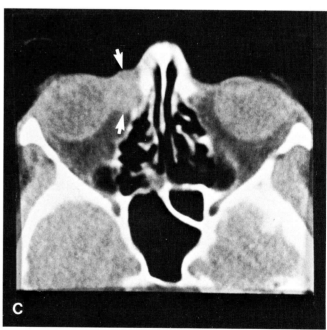

Figures A–C. A soft-tissue mass fills the right nasal cavity and extends back into the nasopharynx. The right nasal lacrimal duct (arrowheads) is enlarged and filled with soft tissue. A small soft-tissue mass (arrows) is also present in the anterior medial right orbit, displacing the globe laterally.*

Follow-up: At surgery, a malignant melanoma was found in the nasal cavity and also within the orbit around the lacrimal sac. A total left maxillectomy with orbital exenteration was done in an attempt to achieve complete resection. Unfortunately, one year later the patient developed abdominal metastases.

Comment: The mass in the inferior meatus of the right nasal cavity extended up the right nasal lacrimal duct to reach the orbit.

*Reprinted from Hesselink JR, New PFJ, Davis KR, et al: Computed tomography of the paranasal sinuses and face: II. Pathological anatomy. J Comput Assist Tomogr 2:569, 1978, with permission.

CASE 8. Nasal Angiofibroma

Two years previously, this 18-year-old male had a transpalatal resection of a nasopharyngeal angiofibroma. Over the past several months, he had progressive right nasal obstruction and intermittent epistaxis. Recently he also noted increased orbital congestion and slight proptosis of the right eye.

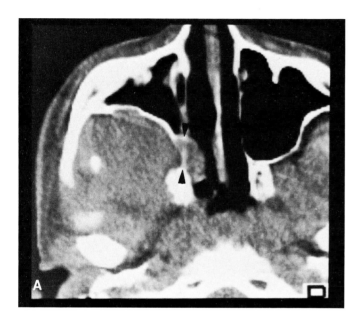

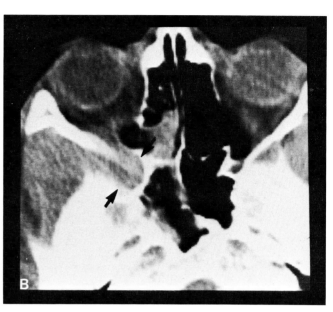

Figure A. An axial scan through the maxillary sinuses reveals a soft-tissue mass in the posterior nasal cavity associated with widening of the pterygopalatine fossa (arrowheads). The mass has extended into the infratemporal fossa and bows the posteror wall of the antrum anteriorly.*

Figure B. A scan through the inferior orbits demonstrates widening of the inferior orbital fissure (arrows).*

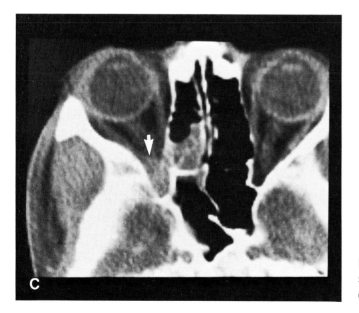

Figure C. On a scan through the midorbits, there is soft-tissue density (white arrow) in the apex of the right orbit.*

Follow-up: The mass was markedly vascular on the angiogram. Following presurgical embolization, a subtotal resection of the angiofibroma was performed.

Comment: A mass in the pterygopalatine fossa or infratemporal fossa can extend superiorly through the inferior orbital fissure to involve the orbit.

Reprinted from Hesselink JR, Weber AL: Pathways of orbital extension of extraorbital neoplasms. J Comput Assist Tomogr 6:596, 1982, with permission.

CASE 9. Carcinoma of the Parotid Gland

This 81-year-old female had carcinoma of the left parotid gland diagnosed 30 years ago, which was treated with surgery and chemotherapy. More recently she developed left proptosis and problems with her left ear.

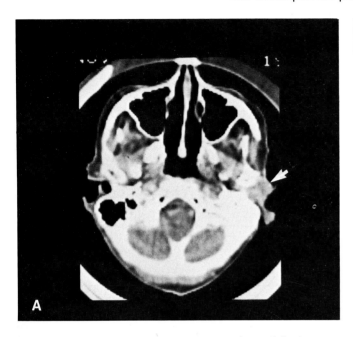

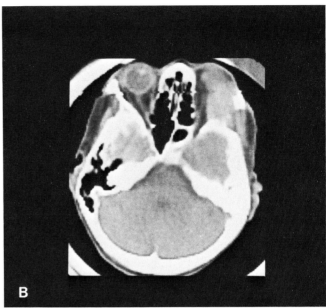

Figure A. There is a soft-tissue mass (arrow) in the region of the left parotid gland. Also noted is opacification of the left mastoid air cells.

Figure B. The mass has extended superiorly to destroy the lateral wall of the left orbit. Soft-tissue mass bulges into the lateral aspect of the orbit.

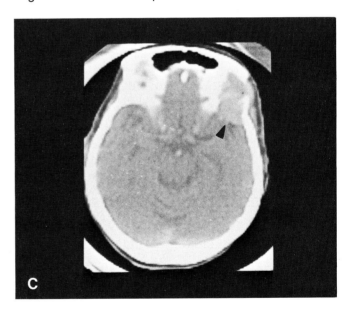

Figure C. The mass has eroded the roof of the orbit and greater wing of the sphenoid to extend into the intracranial cavity (arrowhead).

Follow-up: Radiographic and clinical findings confirmed extension of the parotid tumor to the left ear and orbit.

CASE 10. Meningioma

A 40-year-old female with slowly increasing prominence of the left eye over the past 1½ years. The past few months she had intermittent horizontal diplopia and decreasing visual acuity on the left.

Clinical Findings: Visual acuity was 20/200 OS and 20/30 OD. There was 6 mm of proptosis of the left eye with reduction in orbital resilience. Left optic disc showed mild optic atrophy. Extraocular movements were full.

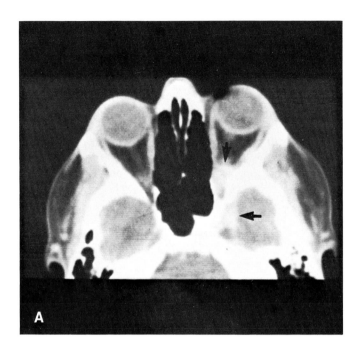
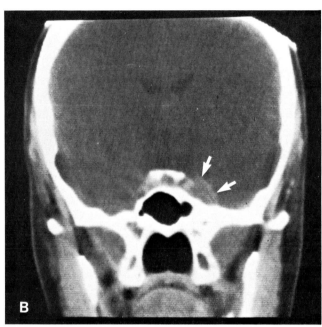

Figures A and B. Axial and coronal scans demonstrate a contrast-enhancing mass in the left paracavernous region and the apex of the left orbit (arrows). Also noted is hyperostosis of the greater sphenoid wing. The left globe is slightly proptotic.

Follow-up: Arteriography revealed a hypervascular mass in the left paracavernous region and orbital apex, as well as some narrowing of the intracavernous carotid artery. A subtotal removal of a medial sphenoid wing meningioma was accomplished through a left frontal craniotomy. The orbit and optic nerve were decompressed. Following surgery her vision in the left eye improved. The residual tumor was treated with radiation therapy.

CASE 11. Meningioma
This is a 41-year-old female with intermittent decreased visual acuity on the left.

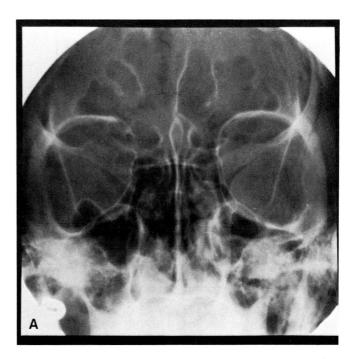

Figure A. A Caldwell view demonstrates sclerosis of the lesser and greater sphenoid wings on the left side with narrowing of the superior orbital fissure.

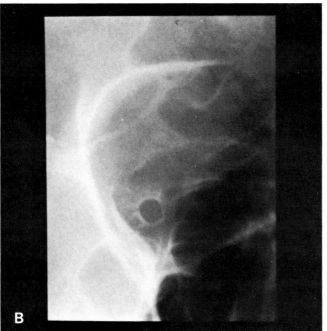

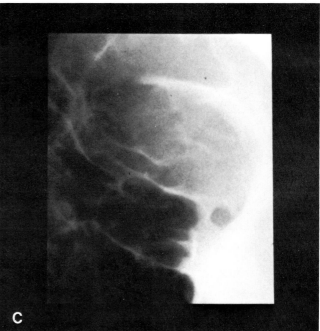

Figures B and C. Rhese views of the right (B) and left (C) optic foramina demonstrate sclerosis about the left optic foramen. The left foramen is also slightly smaller than the right.

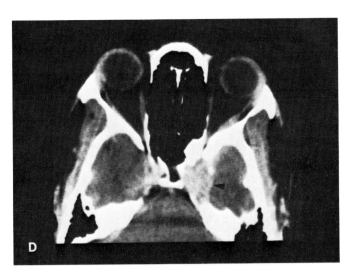
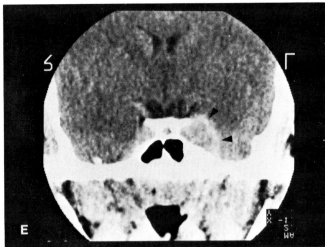

Figures D and E. Coronal and axial scans demonstrate a contrast-enhancing mass (arrowheads) in the left paracavernous area. The mass bulges laterally into the adjacent middle fossa.

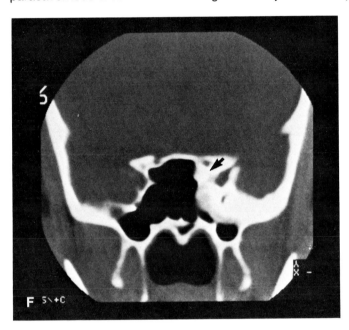

Figure F. A coronal view with a bone window setting demonstrates marked hyperostosis of the floor of the left middle fossa and the adjacent lateral wall of the sphenoid sinus. There is also considerable thickening of the optic strut (arrow).

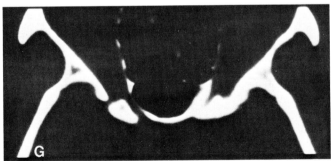
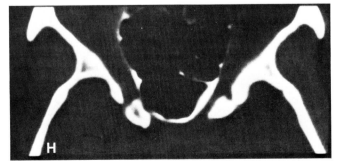

Figures G and H. Axial views of the right (G) and left (H) optic canals show both optic canals to be of about equal caliber, although there is thickening of the bony margins of the left optic canal.

Follow-up: No surgery was done in this case. The radiographic and CT findings are characteristic of meningioma.

CASE 12. Meningioma

A 46-year-old female with a history of prominence of the right eye for 8 years, associated with ptosis and progressive visual loss.

Clinical Findings: Ptosis OD. Marked decrease in visual acuity and limited extraocular movements. Optic atrophy was also noted.

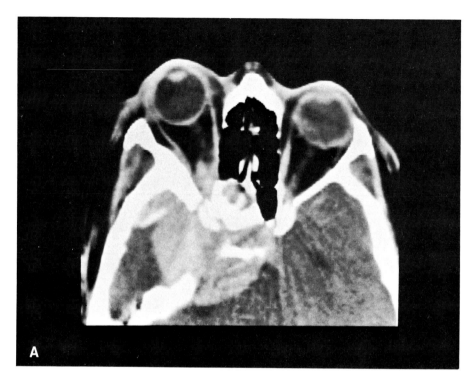

Figure A. Axial scan demonstrates a large contrast-enhancing mass in the right middle fossa and paracavernous regions. The mass has extended into the orbital apex, the sella turcica, and the pontine cisterns on the right side to lie against the brainstem. Also noted is hyperostosis of the sphenoid wing and bony margins of the sphenoid sinus. The right globe is proptotic.

Surgical Findings: At surgery, a right sphenoid wing meningioma was found, which was subtotally removed.

CASE 13. Meningioma

This patient had gradual development of right proptosis over a period of several years.

Clinical Findings: There was 12 mm of exophthalmos OD associated with papilledema. Extraocular movements were full.

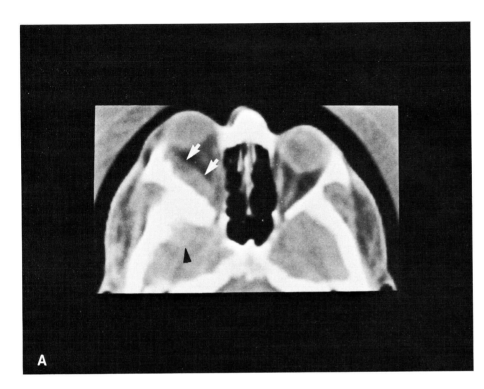

Figure A. There is considerable hyperostosis of the right sphenoid wing. This is associated with a layer of soft tissue against the lateral wall of the right orbit (arrows), as well as a soft-tissue mass in the middle fossa (arrowhead). The right globe is proptotic. The ethmoid and sphenoid sinuses are clear.

Follow-up: At surgery, the roof of the orbit, the pterion, and the posterior wall of the orbit down to the superior orbital fissure were removed. A very thick en plaque meningioma was found, with soft-tissue mass on both the orbital and middle fossa sides of the sphenoid wing. The anterior clinoid was also removed to decompress the optic nerve. The papilledema steadily decreased following surgery.

CASE 14. Meningioma

This is a 49-year-old male with failing vision in the left eye over the past year. He had no orbital pain.

Clinical Findings: There was diplopia on right lateral gaze. Also noted was proptosis and optic disk pallor. No ptosis was evident. Visual acuity was 20/20 OD and 20/200 OS. A central scotoma was present in the left visual field. There was reduced resilience of the left orbit.

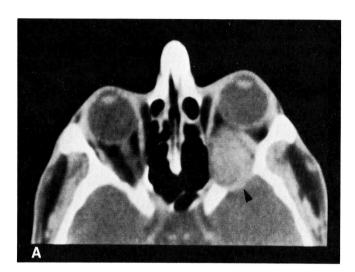 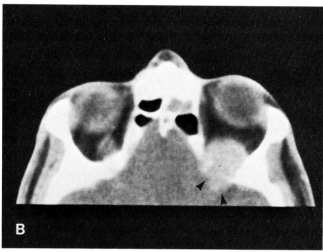

Figures A and B. Axial scans showed a large contrast-enhancing mass in the retrobulbar region of the left orbit. The globe is displaced anteriorly. Also noted is erosion of the sphenoid wing with bulging of the soft-tissue mass into the intracranial cavity (arrowheads).

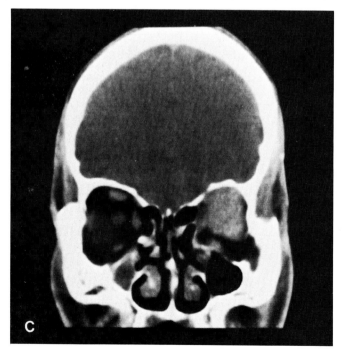 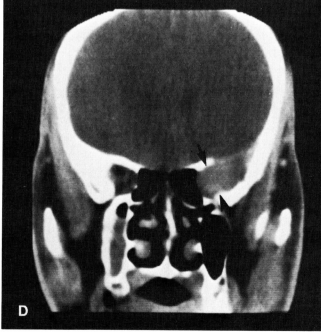

Figures C and D. Coronal scans posterior to the globe further define the mass in the apex of the left orbit. There is marked widening of the superior orbital fissure (arrows). The optic nerve is not clearly defined.

Surgical Findings: At surgery, a meningioma was found attached to the superior orbital fissure. The bulk of the mass was within the orbit and could be dissected free from the orbital structures. Tumor was not attached to the optic nerve. Marked widening of the superior orbital fissure was noted, and the intracranial component of the mass was also removed.

CASE 15. Metastatic Breast Carcinoma

This 50-year-old female first noted some abnormality of her right orbit five months ago, beginning with some puffiness of the eyelids and soreness that progressed to a sunken appearance of the eye and lids. She had no blurring of vision, diplopia, or redness. She had carcinoma of the breast 6 years ago, which was treated by mastectomy and chemotherapy.

Clinical Findings: There was 4 mm of enophthalmos of the right eye. Vision was slightly reduced on that side. There was a sunken appearance to the superior lid sulcus, but no increased orbital resistance or palpable mass. Ocular motility was full. Orbital ultrasound showed a diffuse soft-tissue change involving the retrobulbar fat and extraocular muscles.

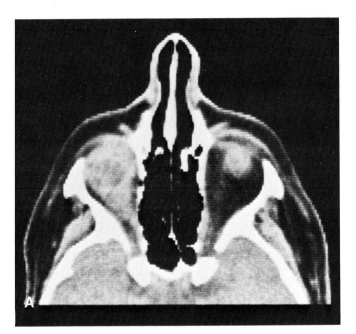 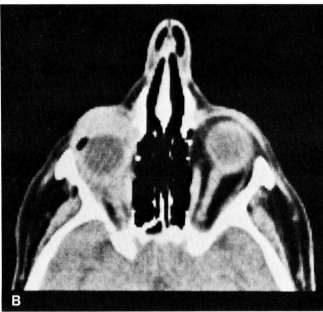

Figures A and B. There is an ill-defined soft-tissue mass involving the anterior soft tissues and the retrobulbar region of the right orbit. The mass is both extraconal and intraconal. The globe is slightly retracted posteriorly into the orbit. The adjacent ethmoid sinuses are clear.

Follow-up: A bone scan revealed multiple areas of increased uptake and bone films confirmed multiple lytic areas, leading to a presumed diagnosis of metastatic breast carcinoma.

Comment: The ill-defined mass in association with enophthalmos in this case is a characteristic appearance of scirrhous carcinoma of the breast metastatic to the orbit.

CASE 16. Metastatic Breast Carcinoma

This is a 58-year-old female with breast carcinoma metastatic to the liver and lungs.

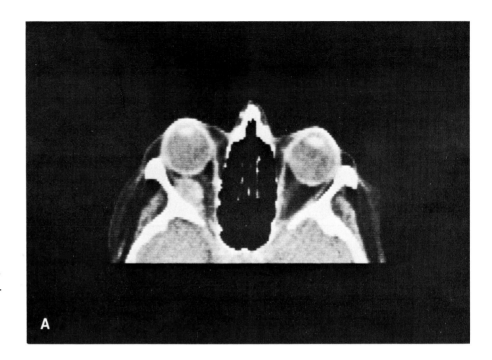

Figure A. There is a soft-tissue mass in the retrobulbar region of the right orbit. The mass appears to infiltrate the lateral rectus muscle and involves both the extraconal and intraconal compartments. No bone destruction is evident. The right globe is proptotic.

Follow-up: In the clinical setting of metastatic breast carcinoma, the orbital lesion was presumed to be a metastasis as well.

CASE 17. Metastatic Scirrhous Carcinoma of the Breast
This is a 62-year-old female who had been treated for carcinoma of the
breast 5 years ago. Axillary nodes were positive at that time.
Physical Examination. Visual acuity was 20/30 OS and 20/25 OD. The patient had slight left enophthalmos, and there was fullness of the upper lid.

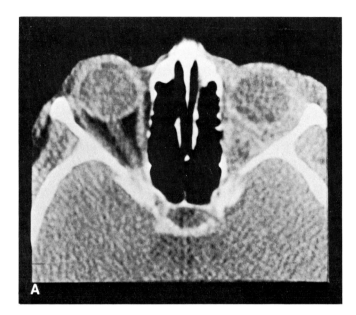 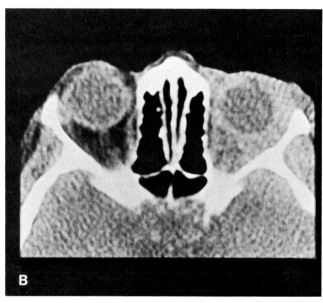

Figures A and B. Axial scans demonstrate an ill-defined mass involving the anterior soft tissues and retrobulbar
structures of the left orbit. The mass appears to be an infiltrative lesion. The left globe is slightly retracted posteriorly into the orbit.*

Follow-up: A biopsy of the upper lid disclosed metastatic scirrhous carcinoma of the breast.

*Reprinted from Hesselink JR, Davis KR, Weber AL, et al: Radiological evaluation of orbital metastases with
emphasis on computed tomography. Radiology 137:365, 1980, with permission.*

CASE 18. Metastatic Breast Carcinoma

This is a 52-year-old female with proptosis of the left eye and diplopia for the past two months. She has no orbital pain.

Clinical Findings: Visual acuity and visual fields were normal. There was 9 mm of proptosis of the left eye. Extraocular movements were severely limited. A large mass was palpable lateral to the globe, and orbital resistance was increased. Orbital ultrasound revealed a large solid tumor in the lateral superior aspect of the left orbit.

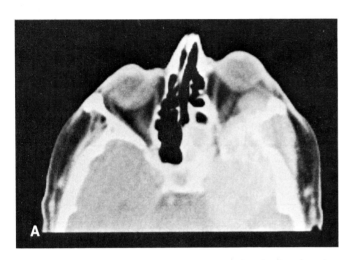

Figure A. Axial scan shows a destructive lesion involving the left sphenoid wing. This is associated with a large soft-tissue mass in the adjacent middle fossa, as well as the temporal fossa and the lateral extraconal space of the left orbit. The globe is markedly proptotic.

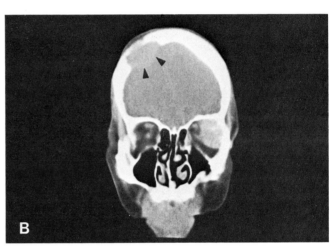

Figure B. A coronal scan through the retrobulbar region further defines a soft-tissue mass in the superior lateral aspect of the left orbit. Also noted is a destructive lesion of the right frontal bone associated with soft-tissue mass (arrowheads).

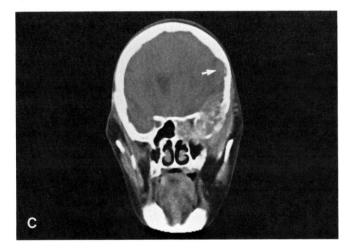

Figure C. A coronal scan at the level of the superior orbital fissures demonstrates the destruction of the sphenoid wing, superior maxilla, and base of sphenoid. A soft-tissue mass is present within the sphenoid sinus and more laterally in the temporal fossa. Also noted is a lytic lesion involving the left frontal bone (white arrow).

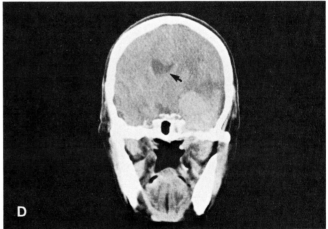

Figure D. A coronal scan through the sella shows the large mass extending superiorly in the left middle fossa associated with some surrounding edema. The lateral ventricles (black arrow) are compressed and displaced to the right.

Follow-up: Additional workup revealed a mass in the left breast and also lytic lesions in two ribs. Biopsy of the breast mass revealed carcinoma of the breast. The patient was treated with a combination of radiation therapy and chemotherapy.

CASE 19. Metastatic Breast Carcinoma

This is a 62-year-old female with widely disseminated metastatic breast carcinoma. She recently developed a left third nerve palsy and retro-orbital pain.

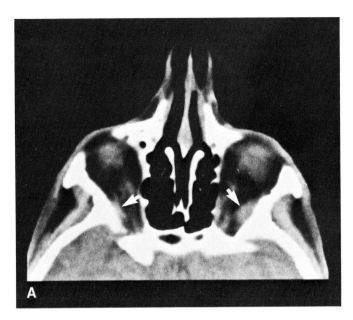

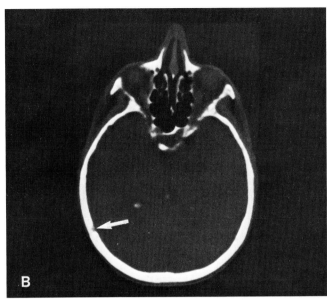

Figure A. An axial scan demonstrates soft-tissue masses in the lateral extraconal spaces of both orbits (arrows).

Figure B. With a bone window setting, there appears to be involvement of the left sphenoid wing and probably the right as well. Also noted is an additional lytic lesion in the calvarium on the right side (arrow).

Follow-up: The patient had multiple additional lytic and blastic lesions, and the abnormalities on the CT scan were presumed to represent metastatic breast carcinoma.

CASE 20. Metastatic Oat Cell Carcinoma of the Larynx

This is a 62-year-old female with oat cell carcinoma of the larynx. A metastatic workup revealed multiple bony metastases.

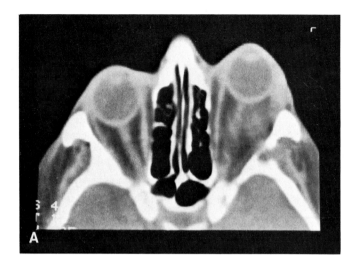 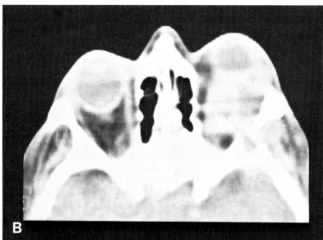

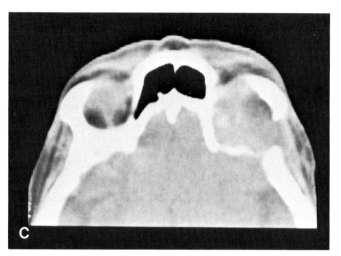

Figures A–C. A series of axial scans shows destruction of the left sphenoid wing and roof of the orbit associated with a large soft-tissue mass in the superior aspect of the orbit. The mass also extends laterally into the temporal fossa. In addition, there is destruction of the floor of the anterior cranial fossa. The left globe is markedly proptotic.

Follow-up: With the other associated findings of disseminated disease, the destructive lesion of the left sphenoid wing and orbit was presumed to represent metastatic oat cell carcinoma of the larynx.

CASE 21. Metastatic Carcinoma of the Prostate

71-year-old male with metastatic carcinoma of the prostate and left proptosis.
Clinical Examination: The soft-tissue mass was palpable in the lateral aspect of the left orbit.

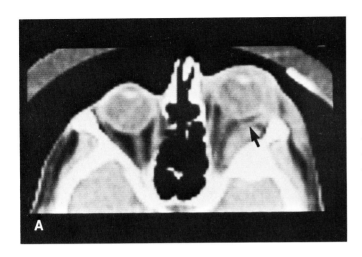

Figure A. An axial scan demonstrates sclerosis and thickening of the left sphenoid wing. This is associated with soft-tissue mass in the lateral extraconal space of the left orbit. The lateral rectus muscle is displaced medially (arrow) and the left globe is proptotic. Also noted is increased soft-tissue density in the anterior lateral aspect of the orbit. The anterior density appears to be separate from the retrobulbar mass.

Follow-up: The anterior soft tissue was thought to be an inflammatory process. Due to the presence of other bone metastases, the sphenoid lesion was presumed to be metastatic carcinoma of the prostate. This was treated with radiation therapy, and a follow-up scan was obtained a few months later.

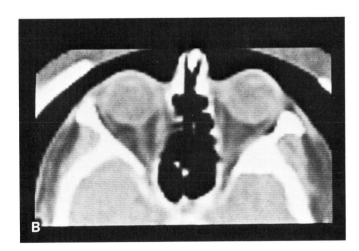

Figure B. The follow-up scan demonstrates resolution of the lateral preseptal mass and also the retrobulbar mass. Again noted is the sclerosis of the left sphenoid wing. The proptosis has partially resolved.

CASE 22. Metastatic Carcinoma of the Prostate
This is a 56-year-old male with carcinoma of the prostate and multiple metastases to the bones and liver. Recently he developed decreasing vision and anosmia.

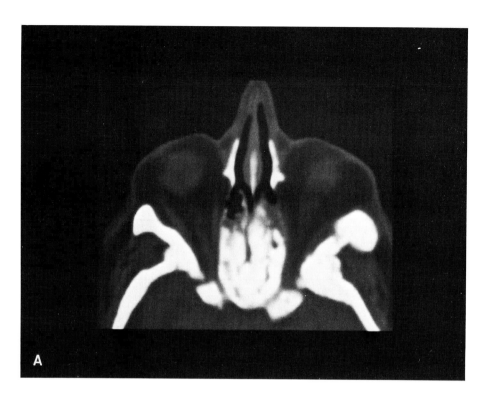

Figure A. There is considerable sclerosis of both sphenoid wings and the sphenoid and ethmoid sinuses. Both optic canals are constricted, particularly on the left side. Also noted is excessive orbital fat bilaterally.

Follow-up: The patient had multiple other osteoblastic metastases, and the changes in the sphenoid and ethmoid sinuses were therefore presumed to be metastatic carcinoma of the prostate. The excessive orbital fat is thought to be related to the patient's steroid therapy.

CASE 23. Metastatic Carcinoma of the Prostate

This is a 69-year-old male with a history of carcinoma of the prostate. In the previous month he had had pain and swelling of the left eye.

Clinical Findings: Left proptosis. He had almost no vision in the left eye, and an inferior temporal field defect was present. Extraocular movements were limited. Orbital ultrasound showed a mass in the posterior lateral aspect of the left orbit associated with some swelling of the optic nerve.

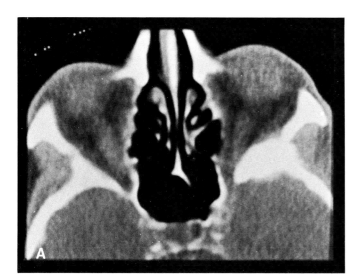 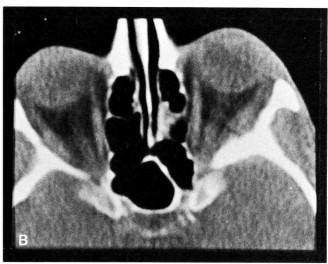

Figures A and B. Axial scans demonstrate sclerosis of the left sphenoid wing associated with some thickening of the soft tissues along the lateral aspect of the orbit. The globe is slightly proptotic.

Follow-up: A metastatic workup revealed no other evidence of metastatic disease. A biopsy of the orbital lesion revealed metastatic carcinoma of the prostate to the left sphenoid wing.

CHAPTER SIX

Vascular Disorders

When considering vascular lesions of the orbit, some authors include capillary and cavernous hemangioma, lymphangioma, and hemangiopericytoma. These lesions usually present as discrete masses and were therefore discussed in Chapter 4 under Primary Orbital Tumors. The vascular abnormalities of concern in this chapter include orbital varices, arteriovenous (AV) malformations, carotid cavernous shunts, and aneurysms. These lesions often cause proptosis but also have other features that distinguish them from tumors. The orbital lesion is often associated with or reflects an extraorbital problem.

ORBITAL VARIX *(Cases 1–3)*

Orbital varices have been classified into primary and secondary types. Primary varices include a congenital variety as well as those that present in middle age. The secondary varices are associated with an AV malformation or carotid-cavernous fistula. The secondary varices are not true venous malformations and are more appropriately discussed under the specific arterial abnormality.

Congenital venous malformations of the orbit or congenital orbital varices result in proptosis soon after birth or in early childhood. They enlarge during childhood but become static after skeletal growth has stopped. About 75 percent have dilated veins on the conjunctiva and within the eyelids. Some also have varices of the forehead, palate, and ipsilateral side of the body. There is an apparent association with Klippel-Trenauney syndrome.[1]

A significant number of orbital varices present in middle age. Hobbs et al.[2] believed these developed from hemangiomas. According to their hypothesis, the original lesion is a capillary hemangioma, which acquires more venous connections to become a cavernous hemangioma. The dilated blood spaces continue to enlarge during life to form varices. Although this is a feasible explanation of why some varices present in middle age, there are no scientific data to confirm this hypothesis.

The classic history of orbital varices is recurrent and intermittent exophthalmos. Any increase in orbital venous pressure results in enlargement of the varix and proptosis. This occurs with crying, coughing, the Valsalva maneuver, bending forward, jugular compression, or extension of the neck. After the episode the eye goes back to normal or there may even be enophthalmos. Recurrent exophthalmos by itself is not specific for a varix and can also occur with lymphangioma, neurofibromatosis, ruptured dermoid, hemorrhage, ethmoiditis, recurrent emphysema from a sinus, and angioneurotic edema. A provocative maneuver to increase orbital venous pressure helps separate out the orbital varix.[3] Recurrent proptosis may be due to thrombosis of varices, resulting in acute inflammation, pain, and swelling.

In a series of 12 cases of congenital orbital varices, Lloyd et al.[4] found that the orbit was enlarged in 8 and phleboliths were present in 6 cases. Phleboliths are formed by venous thrombosis and subsequent calcification. They are also found in hemangiomas, but if phleboliths are seen both within and outside the orbit, they are very likely due to a venous malformation.

Large venous lakes or vascular markings in the ipsilateral frontal bone are often present with an orbital varix.

Arteriography is helpful mainly to exclude an AV malformation. There is usually no arterial abnormality other than vascular displacement, because no direct connections exist between the arterial circulation and the varix. Similarly, the varix frequently is not seen on venous phase, because it is often somewhat isolated from the main venous circulation of the orbit.[4]

Orbital venography is more successful at demonstrating the varix. This can be done with direct puncture of the angular vein or via a forehead vein. Since the veins have no values, the contrast flows freely into all the venous structures of the orbit.[1]

Orbital varices appear as fusiform or globular densities on CT scan. They have smooth, well-defined margins and enhance brightly with contrast. Maneuvers to increase the orbital venous pressure can be used in conjunction with CT to establish the diagnosis. By taking scans before and during a Valsalva maneuver, the orbital varix may be observed to increase in size, confirming the diagnosis.[5] When this phenomenon is observed, venography probably is unnecessary.

Vision is seldom affected by venous malformations because they are under low pressure. Indications for surgery are usually purely cosmetic. Prominent disfiguring veins in the lids or on the sclera can be surgically removed.

ARTERIOVENOUS MALFORMATIONS (Cases 4 and 5)

Arteriovenous malformations of the orbit are rare as isolated lesions and are usually associated with intracranial AV malformations. The Wyburn-Mason syndrome consists of an AV malformation extending from the midbrain along the anterior visual pathways to the orbit and retina. Involvement of the optic tracts, chiasm, and nerve in this condition leads to optic atrophy and gliosis. Angiomatosis of the retina is a feature of von Hippel-Lindau's disease.[3] AV malformations in the anterior orbit may have a traumatic origin.[6]

Orbital AV malformations characteristically produce unilateral pulsatile exophthalmos. The associated bruit is often audible to the patient. Proptosis is usually present, and the retinal vessels are distended and tortuous.[7]

The ophthalmic artery is a prominent arterial contributor to orbital AV malformations. Additional supply is often present from orbital branches of the middle meningeal, internal maxillary, and facial arteries. With pure orbital malformations, the venous drainage is predominantly posterior into the cavernous sinus via the superior and inferior ophthalmic veins. The inferior ophthalmic vein has additional venous connections with the pterygoid plexus. With associated intracranial malformations, the flow in the ophthalmic veins is often reversed and they drain into the anterior facial vein.

Arteriography is the definitive procedure in the evaluation of these lesions. Selective injections into the internal carotid, internal maxillary, middle meningeal, and facial arteries are essential for accurate mapping of the arterial supply. Even if a varix is present, venography may not opacify the varix because of the increased pressure in the arterialized vein.

On CT scan, orbital AV malformations appear as irregular tortuous structures that demonstrate marked contrast enhancement. They are found in both the intraconal and extraconal compartments. If a malformation simulates a mass lesion, a dynamic scan may reveal characteristic rapid AV shunting. Prominence of the ipsilateral cavernous sinus may be evident on CT scan. An intracranial component of a malformation will also be demonstrated.[8,9]

CAROTID-CAVERNOUS FISTULA (Cases 6 and 7)

Carotid-cavernous fistulas can be traumatic or spontaneous. The spontaneous ones are secondary to rupture of an intracavernous carotid aneurysm or a dural AV malformation.[10]

Carotid-cavernous fistulas usually present with rapid onset of orbital congestion and exophthalmos. The exophthalmos is pulsatile in 80 percent and bilateral in 10 percent. Patients often hear a bruit or noise in the head. Severe stretching of the optic nerve may lead to visual loss and even blindness. The increased orbital venous pressure results in elevated intraoccular pressure and dilated conjunctival veins. Pressure within the cavernous sinus or superior orbital fissure can lead to cranial nerve palsies. Usually the sixth nerve is the first affected.[7] Proptosis and an enlarged superior ophthalmic vein are the common findings on CT scan. The vein crosses the orbit above the optic nerve and below the superior rectus muscle. It curves forward and medially from the superior orbital fissure to the trochlea.[9] Weisberg[11] determined the normal diameter of the superior ophthalmic vein to be 2 mm anteriorly and 3.5 mm posteriorly. Any measurement above this may indicate an underlying fistula or malformation. The extraocular muscles may be enlarged due to venous congestion.[12] If the superior ophthalmic vein remains dilated, the superior orbital fissure can enlarge over time. With high-flow fistulas there may be aneurysmal dilatation of the cavernous sinus, which can simulate an enhancing parasellar mass.

ANEURYSMS

Aneurysms of the ophthalmic artery occur most often at the origin from the internal carotid artery. In this location they may simulate a pituitary tumor or present with a subarachnoid hemorrhage. As they enlarge they may produce visual loss or a third nerve palsy. Aneurysms of the intraorbital segment of the ophthalmic artery behave like slow-growing tumors and cause proptosis. Rupture results in an orbital hematoma. Intraorbital aneurysms may coexist with an orbital AV malformation.

Unless they are large, aneurysms at the origin of the ophthalmic artery are difficult to detect on CT scan because of the proximity of the anterior clinoid. Intraorbital aneurysms are rare but should appear as well-defined contrast-enhancing mass lesions.

REFERENCES

1. Wright JE: Orbital vascular anomalies. Trans Am Acad Ophthalmol Otolaryngol 78:606–616, 1974
2. Hobbs HE, DuBoulay GH, Davis RE: Orbital angioma diagnosed by phlebography. Br J Ophthalmol 44:551–557, 1960
3. Jakobiec FA, Jones IS: Vascular tumors, malformations and degenerations. In Jones IS, Jakobiec FA (eds): Diseases of the Orbit. Hagerstown, Md., Harper & Row, 1979, Chap 14
4. Lloyd GA, Wright JE, Morgan G: Venous malformations in the orbit. Br J Ophthalmol 55:505–516, 1971
5. Winter J, Centeno RS, Bentson JR: Maneuver to aid diagnosis of orbital varix by computed tomography. AJNR 2:39–40, 1982
6. Dilenge D: Arteriography in angiomas of the orbit. Radiology 113:355–361, 1974
7. Zizmor J, Lombardi G: Vascular pathology—arterial, arteriovenous and venous. In Zizmor J (ed): Atlas of Orbital Radiography. Birmingham, Aescalapious, 1973, pp 134–151
8. Hilal SK, Trokel SL: Computerized tomography of the orbit using thin sections. Semin Roentgenol 12:137–147, 1977
9. Wende S, Aulich A, Nover A, et al: Computed tomography of orbital lesions. A cooperative study of 210 cases. Neuroradiology 12:123–134, 1977
10. Newton TH, Hoyt WF: Dural arteriovenous shunts in the region of the cavernous sinuses. Neuroradiology 1:71–81, 1971
11. Weisberg LA: Computed tomographic findings in carotid-cavernous fistula. Comput Tomogr 5:31–36, 1981
12. Merrick R, Latchaw RE, Gold LH: Computerized tomography of the orbit in carotid-cavernous fistulae. Comput Tomogr 4:127–132, 1980

CASE 1. Orbital Varix
This patient presented with intermittent exophthalmos.

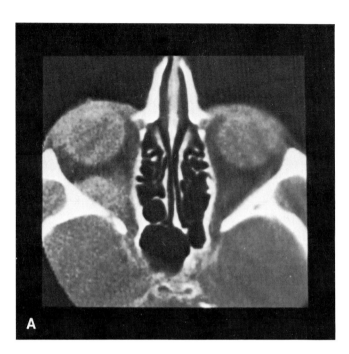 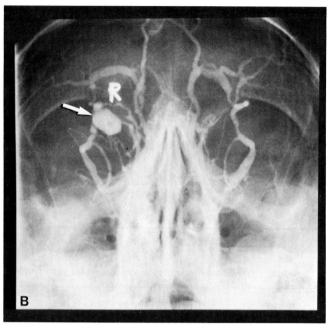

Figure A. An axial scan demonstrates a smoothly marginated mass in the posterior lateral aspect of the right orbit. The globe is slightly proptotic.

Figure B. An orbital venogram demonstrates an enlarged venous structure (arrow), which is characteristic of an orbital varix.

CASE 2. Orbital Varix

This patient is a 17-year-old male with pain and bulging of the left eye for 3 years. The proptosis was increased by straining, leaning forward, or with a Valsalva maneuver.

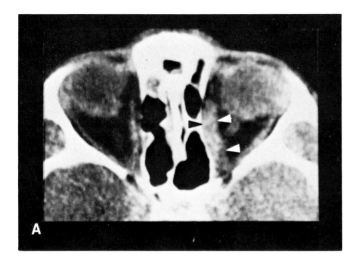 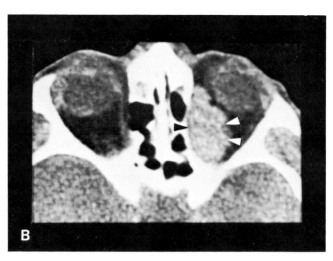

Figure A. A contrast scan demonstrates an elongated mass (arrowheads) in the medial left orbit, which parallels the medial rectus muscle. Medial bowing of the lamina papyracea indicates that the mass has been there for a long time.*

Figure B. A scan done during a Valsalva maneuver shows marked enlargement of the mass (arrowheads). The proptosis is also increased.*

Follow-up: The enlargement of the mass with a Valsalva maneuver is diagnostic of an orbital varix. Since the symptoms were relatively minor, no surgery was recommended at this time.

Reprinted from Winter J, Centeno RS, Bentson JR: Maneuver to aid diagnosis of orbital varix by computed tomography. AJNR 2:39–40, © 1982, with permission.

CASE 3. Orbital Varix

A 55-year-old female with proptosis of the right eye. She had several episodes of spontaneous orbital hemorrhage during childhood but had no problem with her vision. The proptosis persisted into adult life, but otherwise she has been asymptomatic.

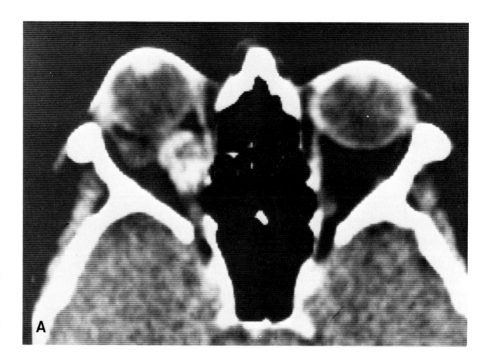

Figure A. CT scan shows a contrast-enhancing mass in the medial intraconal compartment of the right orbit. The globe is slightly proptotic. The nonenhancing areas of the mass probably represent thrombosis.*

Diagnosis: Orbital ultrasonography was also compatible with an orbital varix. The combination of history and findings on the diagnostic studies is most compatible with orbital varix.

Reprinted from Krohel G: Orbital Disease. New York, Grune & Stratton, 1981, p 72, with permission.

CASE 4. Arteriovenous Malformation

This 57-year-old female was in good health until six months ago, when she noted the onset of ptosis of the right eyelid, intermittent diplopia, and proptosis. She also wakes up in the morning with a throbbing pain behind the right eye. She can see out of the eye, but there is a gray film. The past few months she has also noted a "swishing sound" near her right ear. She had no history of trauma.

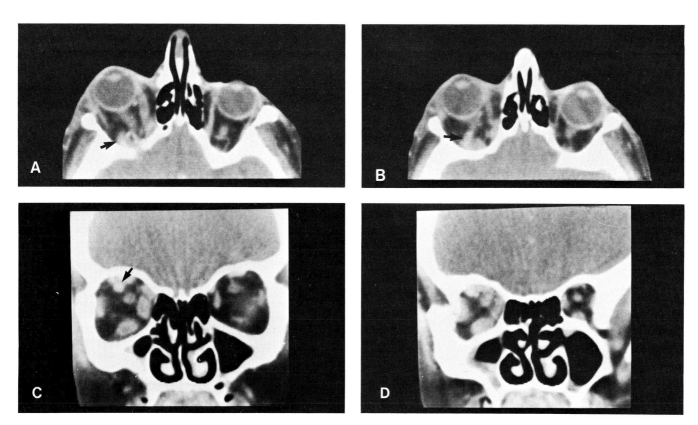

Figures A–D. The right globe is moderately proptotic. The superior ophthalmic vein (small arrows) is enlarged and enhanced on these contrast scans. On the coronal scans, it is positioned superior and lateral to the optic nerve just below the superior rectus muscle. All of the extraocular muscles of the right orbit are enlarged.

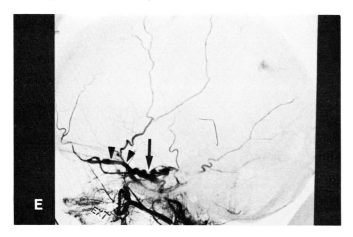

Figure E. The external carotid arteriogram demonstrates a dural AV malformation (large arrow) in the region of the cavernous sinus. There is AV shunting into the cavernous sinus and opacification of the superior ophthalmic vein (arrowheads).

Comment: The AV shunt results in increased pressure in the cavernous sinus and orbital veins. The enlargement of the extraocular muscles is due to venous congestion.

CASE 5. Facial Angioma

This 40-year-old female had a massive congenital hemangioma of the left side of the face. Clinically, the hemangioma involved the eyelids, soft palate, and pharynx.

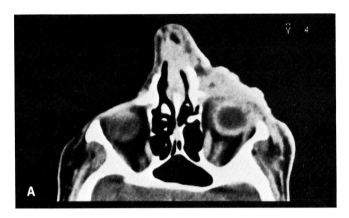

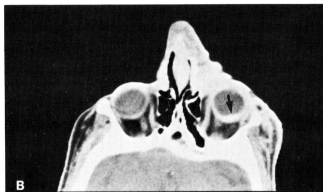

Figures A–C. Axial scans demonstrate an extensive irregular, enhancing mass in the subcutaneous tissues of the left side of the face. It extends into the nasal septum and involves the anterior structures of the orbit. It also involves the retrobulbar structures of the left orbit more superiorly (C). In B, there is thickening and enhancement of the posterior lateral aspect of the choroid of the left eye (arrow), consistent with choroid angioma.

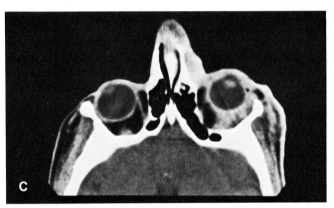

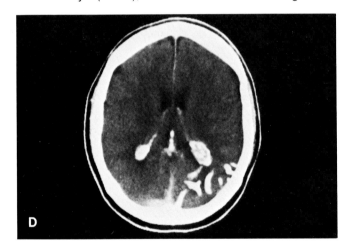

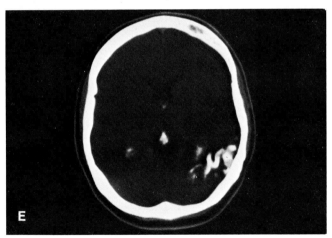

Figures D and E. Axial sections through the brain show angiomatous lesions involving the left occipital and posterior temporal lobes, as well as the glomus of the choroid plexus of the left lateral ventricle.

Surgical Findings: The facial angiomatous lesion was partially removed. Histologic examination revealed both capillary hemangioma (port wine stain) and also elements of cavernous hemangioma within the deeper regions of the face. Angiomatous lesions of the left choroid were noted on fundoscopic examination. The patient had Sturge-Weber syndrome.

CASE 6. Carotid-cavernous Fistula
This 82-year-old female was in a motor vehicle accident and sustained a concussion and contusions to both orbits. A few days after the accident, she noted a noise in the head and developed double vision. Clinical examination revealed proptosis of the right eye, subconjunctival hemorrhage, and a total ophthalmoplegia of the right eye. Vision was normal.

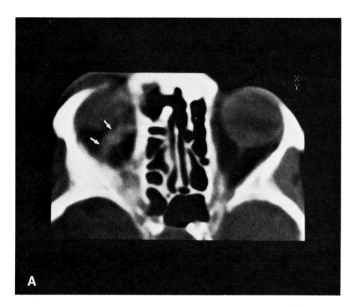

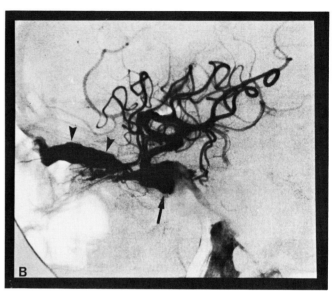

Figure A. CT scan shows an enlarged and tortuous superior ophthalmic vein (arrows) coursing obliquely through the intraconal compartment of the right orbit. It lies above the optic nerve. On lower sections, the globe was proptotic.

Figure B. A lateral carotid arteriogram demonstrates a carotid-cavernous fistula with early filling of the cavernous sinus (arrow). The superior ophthalmic vein (arrowheads) is markedly enlarged.

CASE 7. Carotid-cavernous Fistula

This 19-year-old female was in a motorcycle accident 2 years ago, which resulted in multiple skull and facial fractures, cerebral contusions, and multiple chest and abdominal injuries. She was in coma for three weeks, which was followed by posttraumatic psychosis. She had intermittent frontal headaches since then, but in the past three to four months she began "hearing her headaches." On physical examination, she had left proptosis with a left sixth nerve palsy. A loud bruit was also heard over the left eye.

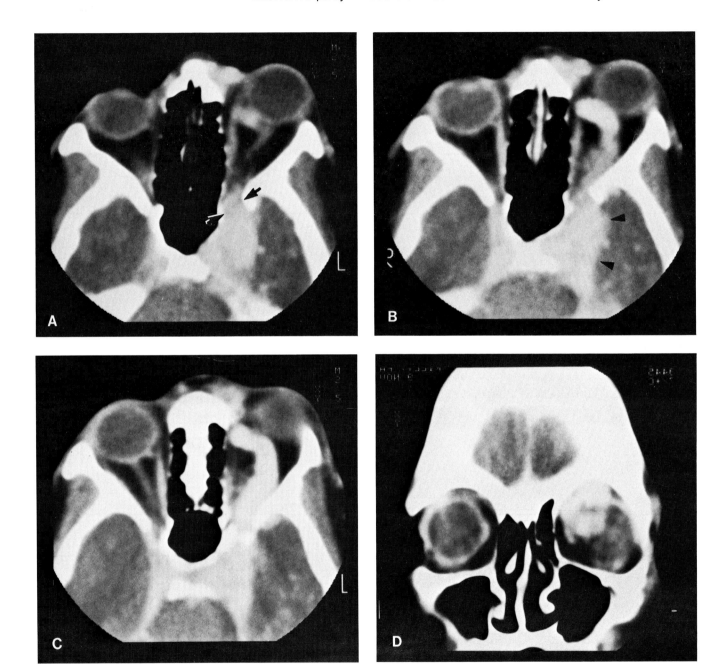

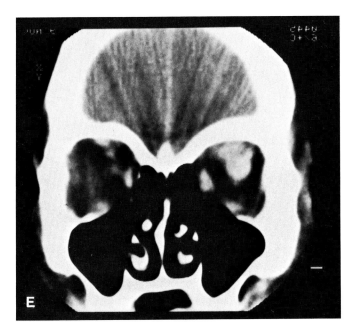

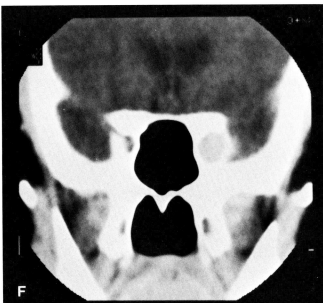

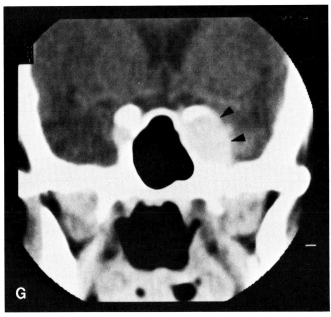

Figures A–G. Axial and coronal scans demonstrate a markedly enlarged and tortuous left superior ophthalmic vein. Also noted are some prominent vascular structures in the anterior medial and superior aspects of the orbit (B and D). These findings are associated with a homogeneously enhancing left parasellar mass (arrowheads), which represents aneurysmal dilatation of the cavernous sinus. The enlarged venous structures have resulted in widening of the superior orbital fissure (arrows). There is erosion of the left side of the dorsum sella (C) and undercutting of the anterior clinoid process (G). Figure E shows slight enlargement of the medial and superior rectus muscles.

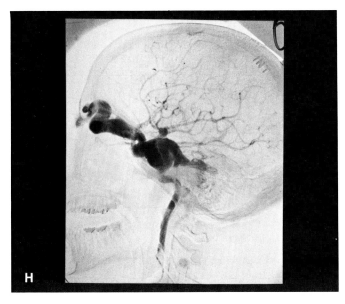

Figure H. A lateral view of the carotid arteriogram demonstrates a carotid-cavernous fistula with marked dilatation of the cavernous sinus. There is prominent venous drainage anteriorly through the superior ophthalmic vein and posteriorly through the superior petrosal sinus.

CHAPTER SEVEN

Inflammatory Disease

This chapter deals with the most frequent causes of exophthalmos. Collectively, inflammatory disease accounts for well over 50 percent of cases of proptosis. Included here is a discussion on infectious orbital cellulitis; the nonorganismal inflammations, which include idiopathic inflammatory pseudotumor and Graves' disease, are also discussed. In view of the close similarities between pseudotumor and lymphoma in their CT appearances, examples of the latter are included in the illustrations for comparison.

ORBITAL CELLULITIS *(Cases 1–16)*

Orbital cellulitis is an acute bacterial infection that can spread from an infection of the paranasal sinuses or eyelid (secondary to trauma, insect bite, or impetigo).[1-4] Much less commonly it can be secondary to hematogenous spread, infection from a retained foreign body, or spread from an infected tooth or middle ear.

Anatomic Considerations

The ethmoid sinus is the earliest to develop, and therefore, acute ethmoiditis with subsequent orbital involvement occurs most frequently in the pediatric age group. This is due primarily to the anatomic contiguity of the structures. The orbital plate of the ethmoid bone, the lamina papyracea, is a thin bone serving as a boundary between the ethmoid sinus and the orbit. Congenital dehiscences in the bone, open suture lines, and the anterior and posterior ethmoidal foramina present numerous potential access routes for sinus inflammation to spread into the orbit.

The complex venous drainage system of the orbit and paranasal sinus undoubtedly also plays a role in the spread of infection. These valveless veins allow free communication with the facial, nasal, and pterygoid venous plexuses. The superior ophthalmic vein anastomoses with the angular vein of the face, allowing facial infection distant from the eyelids to spread posteriorly to the orbit. The inferior ophthalmic vein communicates with venous tributaries from the lacrimal sac, eyelids, pterygoid venous plexus, and the maxillary antrum. There is a rich plexus of veins surrounding the nasolacrimal duct communicating with the plexuses of the turbinates, linings of the sinuses, and the veins of the orbit.[5]

The evolution of the spread of orbital cellulitis is also influenced by the integrity of the components of the orbital fascia, specifically the periorbita and orbital septum. The periorbita is the periosteal lining of the orbit, and it represents an important soft-tissue barrier between the sinuses and the orbital contents. It is a tough fibrous membrane but can easily be stripped from bone, except at suture sites. This periosteum may block the spread of infection but at the price of a subperiosteal abscess. The development of such an abscess can readily elevate the periorbita, displacing it into the orbit.

The orbital septum is a membranous sheath arising as a reflection of the periorbita at the orbital rim and extending circumferentially to insert into the upper and lower tarsal plates[6,7] (see Chapter 1, Fig. 7, 8, and 10). The soft tissues anterior to the orbital septum constitute the preseptal space and inflammations of this space are termed preseptal or periorbital cellulitis. Deep to the septum and confined within the periorbita is the orbit proper, and inflammations of this space represent true orbital cellulitis. The orbital septum is tough and resistant, also functioning as a barrier to the transmission of inflammation. There are no lymph nodes or lymphatic channels in the orbit.

Pathogenesis

The development of orbital cellulitis as a complication of acute sinusitis progresses through several stages.[8] Initially, there is impedance in the drainage of the superior ophthalmic vein into the congested ethmoid vessels due to elevated pressure within the ethmoid labyrinth. This restriction of flow results in an inflammatory edema with swelling of the eyelids, with or without orbital swelling. At this stage, there is no limitation of extraocular movement and vision is normal. Slight proptosis may be present, the result of edema of the orbital contents.

The next stage involves actual inflammatory infiltrate with inflammatory cells and bacteria spreading rapidly through the orbital fat, which offers little resistance. This results in diffuse orbital edema and a true orbital cellulitis. Unchecked, this can rapidly progress into an orbital abscess. Abscess formation is accompanied by exophthalmos, chemosis, ophthalmoplegia, and severe compromise of vision. The pus can rupture through the septum, draining anteriorly through the eyelid. Extension of phlebitis posteriorly can result in a cavernous sinus thrombosis. This dreaded complication manifests with bilateral ocular signs in a toxic patient. Other rare complications in neglected cases include epidural or brain abscess, meningitis, osteomyelitis, optic neuritis, and blindness.

The stage of orbital cellulitis may not be reached if the periorbita is able to restrict the spread of infection. A subperiosteal abscess may develop with the collection of pus located between the periorbita and orbital wall. This usually indicates advanced suppuration in the contiguous ethmoid labyrinth or frontal sinus.

CT Manifestations

The acute onset of periorbital inflammation in a febrile child frequently presents diagnostic and therapeutic challenges to the clinician. It is important to distinguish an inflammatory process involving the preseptal or periorbital area from a true orbital cellulitis, in view of the greater severity and potential complications of the latter. The clinical evaluation of such patients may be misleading. Inflamed edematous eyelids are common to both, and sometimes it may be impossible to make an adequate evaluation of globe motility, degree of proptosis, and visual acuity in the presence of tense eyelid swelling. The consequences of inadequate treatment are potentially catastrophic, and it is imperative that the full extent of the disease process is recognized early and treated appropriately.

CT of the orbit has established itself as an extremely useful adjunct in the diagnosis and management of the spectrum of orbital cellulitis and its complications.[9–12] In the first instance, CT usually determines the underlying cause of the orbital inflammation. The presence of sinus pathology is confirmed by the demonstration of opacification and/or air-fluid levels in the involved air spaces. Occasionally, an intraorbital foreign body may be identified as the offending agent.[13]

CT can clearly distinguish preseptal involvement from true orbital cellulitis. In the former, the edematous thickening of the eyelid with obliteration of its normal fat planes is readily apparent. The sharp transition of the swollen tissues with the normal-appearing postseptal structures at the level of the orbital septum is clearly visualized.

In the development of the inflammatory infiltrate of true orbital cellulitis, early scanning will initially reveal changes in the fat body. The overall density of the fat increases slightly, often accompanied by small stippled densities. This subtle change is best appreciated with wide window settings and comparison with the contralateral normal orbit. This is followed by the development of more discreet densities as the orbital cellulitis progresses. In most cases, the cellulitis is largely confined to the extraconal space,[12] but unchecked, it enters the muscle cone and may compromise the optic nerve directly. Not infrequently, there is thickening of an extraocular muscle, usually the medial rectus, which indicates a myositis secondary to involvement with the inflammatory process. Invariably with orbital cellulitis, there is concomitant preseptal involvement as well.

The diagnosis of orbital abscess is more difficult. One possible limitation of CT may turn out to be in accurately diagnosing the early development of an intraorbital abscess. The role of contrast enhancement in the diagnosis of orbital abscess remains unclear. In one report, there were three different enhancement patterns—homogeneous, heterogeneous, and ring enhancement, with the homogeneous being the most frequent.[13] More experience with orbital abscess and enhancement patterns is necessary before any definite conclusions can be drawn. It is our impression that any localized intraorbital inflammatory mass, regardless of the enhancement pattern, should be considered suspicious for abscess development, especially if accompanied by a deteriorating clinical picture. The presence of gas bubbles in an inflammatory process is unequivocal evidence of abscess formation.

A subperiosteal abscess typically follows an ethmoiditis and manifests between the periorbita and lamina papyracea. Subperiosteal abscess may form along the orbital roof, usually following frontal sinusitis. Any unusual superior orbital density on axial scanning must be followed by coronal views for more precise localization. A subperiosteal abscess in its early stages will manifest as a small soft-tissue density contiguous with the bony wall. The adjacent extraocular muscle is displaced away from the wall, but there is preservation of a thin extraconal fat plane between the displaced muscle and the soft-tissue density. This confirms that the process is subperiosteal. In more advanced cases, a large subperiosteal abscess compresses the muscle cone without visible fat planes. Contrast administration will enhance the inflamed displaced periorbita. Not infrequently, a mixed picture of subperiosteal abscess and orbital cellulitis is present. A subperiosteal abscess can resolve with vigorous conservative treatment, monitoring the patient carefully. Any progression of symptoms, or even failure to improve, requires immediate surgical drainage.

In summary, CT examination provides an early determination of orbital involvement of an acute inflammatory process. Because of the inherent limitations of the clinical evaluation, a rational form of therapy can be instituted based on the CT demonstration of the precise localization, extent, and progression of the disease process.

IDIOPATHIC INFLAMMATORY PSEUDOTUMOR (Cases 17–24)

Pseudotumor is a restricted category of nonspecific inflammation of the orbit without identifiable cause. This definition therefore excludes specific infectious, granulomatous, and collagen-vascular disorders. Thus, inflammations caused by foreign bodies, amyloid, parasites, bacteria, fungi, ruptured dermoid cysts, Graves' disease, sarcoid, tuberculosis, syphilis, and well-defined vasculitides such as polyarteritis nodosa and Wegener's granulomatosis should be recognized as such and not included as part of the syndrome of idiopathic inflammatory pseudotumor.[14]

Incidence
The condition is rare, but may amount to about one-quarter of cases with unilateral exophthalmos.[15] Males and females are equally affected. This is in contrast to thyroid ophthalmopathy, in which there is female predominance. There is no racial predilection, and the disease occurs more commonly in middle age, although it may manifest in children and adolescents, as well as the elderly.

Clinical Manifestations
Pseudotumor usually presents with sudden onset of painful proptosis with swelling of the lids, conjunctival edema, and decreased ocular motility in a patient with considerable malaise. On palpation, a hard mass is often found in the orbit.[16] The course of the disease may be remitting, in which the inflammation may spontaneously regress or respond to steroids. A chronic progressive course lasting many years despite treatment is also characteristic. The disease tends to be unilateral. Bilaterality would suggest an underlying systemic disease or endocrine exophthalmos.

Pathologic Features
The inflammatory infiltrate may be localized into a tumoral form or establish itself in a diffuse pattern with no distinct mass. The histologic picture varies between lymphocytic infiltrates, granulomatous formation, vasculitis, or a dense collagen or hyalinization pattern. There may be isolated organ involvement such as a myositis or dacryoadenitis. In such cases even the histoloic differentiation with Graves' disease and Sjogren syndrome, respectively, may be difficult. When a myositis is present, the inferior rectus is most frequently involved, either alone or with other muscles.

One important histologic variant of pseudotumor, benign lymphocytic hyperplasia, deserves special mention. The cellular infiltrate in this subgroup is composed of monomorphous mature lymphocytes and is felt by some authors to be a possible forerunner of lymphoma.[14] Other authors, however, state that few lymphomas begin in the orbit.[17] The issue is further confused, as in as many as 40 percent of patients, the histologic diagnosis of pseudotumor versus lymphoma is incorrect.[18] A long-term follow-up may be needed for definitive diagnosis, since those patients who eventually do develop systemic lymphoma do so after an average of four years.[18] This opinion is somewhat at variance with the earlier impression that there is no difference among the histologic groups as far as the symptomatology, clinical course, or prognosis is concerned, and that they are all probably only various stages of one disease.[16] This conviction is probably incorrect, however, as immunohistologic techniques have only recently improved differentiation among the subgroups. Three cases of lymphoma are included in this chapter to demonstrate the similarities with pseudotumor in their CT appearances (Cases 25–27).

CT Manifestations
The CT appearance of orbital pseudotumor reveals a broad range of pathologic changes. Although the findings may often be very suggestive of idiopathic inflammatory pseudotumor, they are by no means specific. Depending on the pattern of involvement, differentiation from an orbital tumor, Graves' disease, lymphoma, sarcoid, or other specific granulomas, or even an orbit neoplasm with sinus extension, may not be possible.

The pseudotumor mass may appear as an isolated discreet lesion with well-defined borders resembling any orbital mass such as a neoplasm or specific granuloma.[13] The inflammatory changes can be confined to the region of the globe, resulting in an apparent thickening of the scleral margin. This appearance of a thickened wall of the globe is usually not an isolated finding, but occurs in association with soft-tissue involvement of the adjacent optic nerve, muscles, lacrimal gland, or fat body.[19] The soft-tissue densities have a predilection for involvement of the posterior globe.[20]

The thickened rim of the globe probably represents some inflammation of the sclera,[21] with a significant contribution due to a tenonitis with pooling of fluid in Tenon's space.[22] Certainly ultrasound examination has demonstrated an effusion in Tenon's space in such cases, and it would appear that the predominating lesion is in fact a periocular inflammation, which accounts for the apparent thickened sclera.

A thickened scleral margin together with a localized discreet mass abutting the posterior globe should, in fact, arouse suspicions for a lurking lymphoma.[23] Even though the lesion may be steroid-responsive, satisfying criteria for diagnosing pseudotumor, these patients should be worked up for lymphoma, including close observation for the development of systemic manifestations over a number of years.

Scleral enhancement with contrast administration has been reported to occur in about 50 percent of cases.[21] The major contribution to this apparent thickening of the scleral rim is involvement of Tenon's capsule[23] and is not specific for pseudotumor. Identical changes are found in lymphoma and sarcoid, making distinction impossible on CT alone. Similarly, following trauma, postoperatively, and in acute orbital cellulitis, thickening of the margin of the globe may also occur. In these cases, however, the underlying clinical background is more obvious.

Orbital pseudotumor can violate the orbital wall and present as a simultaneous mass in the orbit and adjacent ethmoid sinus.[24] This picture conforms much more to that of a malignant tumor with invasion, with the correct diagnosis only being made by biopsy.

Pseudotumor localized to extraocular muscle involvement may mimic Graves' disease in several respects. In our experience, the configuration of the muscle thickening appears identical in most cases to that of endocrine ophthalmopathy. Other authors, however, have indicated that the muscular enlargement in pseudotumor is less regular than in Graves' disease.[25]

Myositic pseudotumor is usually uniocular and usually involves only one muscle, commonly the inferior rectus. Graves' disease, on the other hand, most frequently reveals bilateral involvement, despite unilateral symptoms. In addition, usually several muscles in each orbit are involved. There is, however, some overlap between these two entities, and distinguishing one from the other may be very difficult in view of the fact that thyroid ophthalmopathy may manifest in a euthyroid patient and occasionally be unilateral. It is estimated that unilateral Graves' disease occurs in 2 to 5 percent of cases, whereas bilateral pseudotumor involvement occurs in 10 to 15 percent of cases.[21]

Sometimes the myositic pseudotumor will have associated multifocal changes other than in muscle that allow a diagnosis of pseudotumor to be made with relative confidence. Infiltrative changes in the adjacent fat, associated periocular involvement, or a separate discreet mass, together with a thickened muscle, all favor pseudotumor. Bilateral orbital pseudotumor should arouse suspicions of an underlying systemic disorder.

The myositic form of pseudotumor should probably be distinguished from other forms of pseudotumor and recognized as a distinct clinical entity. Suppression and resolution of the myositis occur more readily with steroids than in other types of pseudotumor.[19,25] The myositis may, in fact, resolve spontaneously without any treatment.

Varying degrees of contrast enhancement of the abnormal soft tissue are seen in most cases of pseudotumor. This, however, does not reveal previously undetected areas of involvement, and no additional information is obtained.[19,20]

CT is an excellent method for monitoring the response to steroid therapy in pseudotumor,[26] since the diminution of the abnormal soft-tissue mass with concomitant increasing definition of the contiguous normal structures is readily appreciated. In the absence of clinical information, acute and chronic pseudotumor cannot be differentiated by CT alone, unless serial studies have been obtained.[19]

GRAVES' DISEASE *(Cases 28–36)*

Incidence

Endocrine ophthalmopathy in adults is the most common cause of either unilateral or bilateral proptosis, accounting for approximately 16 percent of patients presenting with unilateral proptosis,[27] and the great majority of cases of bilateral proptosis. The orbitopathy of Graves' disease may occur before, during, or after the phase of systemic hyperthyroidism. It most frequently manifests in middle-aged females, with an overall female-to-male preponderance of 4:1. It may occur in children, accounting for 14 percent of all causes of proptosis in children under 15 years of age.[28] In almost all patients who present with unilateral Graves' exophthalmos, there is subclinical disease in the contralateral "normal" orbit.[25]

Extraocular muscle thickening is reported to be bilaterally symmetrical in 70 percent of cases. It is asymmetrical, either unilaterally or bilaterally in 30 percent of cases.[29] Pure unilateral disease occurs in about 6 percent of cases. The inferior and medial rectus muscles are the most frequently involved, and they are also the most severely affected.

Pathologic Features

The prime abnormality in the orbit appears to be an abundance of mucopolysaccharides (hyaluronic acid), collagen, and glycoproteins, due to hypersecretion of the fibroblasts.[14] The hyaluronic acid has a considerable capacity for binding water, thereby increasing the osmotic pressure of the orbit. Early on, there is a chronic inflammatory infiltrate involving the muscles, fat, and optic nerve. The fat content may increase considerably, but in the late stages it decreases as fibrous tissue is laid down replacing the orbital fat and muscles.

The focus of the insult appears to be mediated through the fibroblast. The underlying mechanism—whether hormonal, antibody, autoimmune, or cell-mediated—remains unresolved.[14] In severe cases, the extraocular muscles may demonstrate an eightfold increase in size, and orbital bulk may increase fourfold.[30] It is postulated that localized swelling at the orbital apex may result in compression of the arterial supply to the optic nerve, resulting in loss of vision.

CT Manifestations

In most cases, the determination of extraocular muscle enlargement is readily apparent. The typical case of Graves' disease will reveal multiple muscle involvement in both orbits. In addition, there may be an increased amount of orbital fat, displacing the orbital septum forwards. If the patient has been treated on prolonged steroid therapy, steroid-induced exophthalmos due to excess fat should be a consideration as well.[31]

The difficulty arises when there is only apparent single-muscle enlargement. One should establish initially that this is not a spurious finding secondary to head rotation, lateral gaze, or nerve palsy (see Chapter 2, Figs. 8 and 9). Minimal muscle enlargement is difficult to determine on CT. Precise measurements of the muscles have been attempted with ultrasonography.[32] However, in view of the fusiform configuration of the muscles and the other variables mentioned above, measurements are probably of little value in distinguishing minimal enlargement from the norm on an axial view. Coronal views are required to evaluate the extraocular muscles fully. Another important indication to perform coronal views is in the determination of an apical orbital mass, which can be mimicked by enlarged extraocular muscles.[33] In the late stages of Graves' ophthalmopathy (Class 5 and 6),[30] CT may detect optic nerve thickening. Finally, bone erosion of the orbit has been reported, presumably as a result of direct pressure from large extraocular muscles.[34]

In summary, CT is not usually necessary for the diagnosis of Graves' disease, but this modality is most useful in patients who present with unilateral proptosis due to endocrine ophthalmopathy, but in whom no clinical or hormonal. evidence of Graves' disease is found.

Differential Diagnosis of Enlarged Extraocular Muscles[25]

1. Graves' disease (see Chapter 7, Figs. 28 to 36).
2. Idiopathic inflammatory pseudotumor (myositis). This is typically characterized by a single isolated enlarged muscle in a patient with acute onset of proptosis with pain on motion of the eye. Response to steroids is good (see Chapter 7, Cases 17, 23, 24).
3. Arteriovenous malformation or carotid-cavernous fistula. In this instance, the CT typically demonstrates a dilated superior ophthalmic vein with diffuse uniform enlargement of all the extraocular muscles in the involved orbit if the shunt is sufficiently large (see Chapter 6, Case 4). The mechanism of enlargement of the muscles is secondary to increased venous pressure, with congestion and swelling of the muscles.
4. Tumor associated with muscle enlargement usually results from muscle invasion or infiltration or by compression with obstruction of venous flow by a strategically located mass (see Chapter 3, Case 17; Chapter 5, Case 16; and Chapter 7, Case 25).
5. Swelling of muscles, usually the medial rectus, in orbital cellulitis (see Chapter 7, Cases 6, 7, 9–12).
6. Acute extraocular muscle hematoma has also been reported.[32] This may be spontaneous or trauma-induced.
7. Spurious muscle enlargements (see Chapter 2, Figs. 8 and 9; and Chapter 7, Case 26).

SPECIFIC CHRONIC INFLAMMATORY DISEASES (Cases 37–39)

A number of chronic inflammatory and granulomatous conditions resulting from specific identifiable infections or etiologies can involve the orbit. The list is extensive[14] and includes sarcoidosis, amyloidosis, Wegener's granulomatosis, fungal and parasitic diseases, tuberculosis, and the histiocytoses.[35–57] Reports of CT findings in these disorders are sparse or nonexistent, but will in time, no doubt, appear. We have encountered sarcoidosis and mucormycosis in our case material, and we include brief descriptions of these disorders and others in which there have been CT reports.

Sarcoidosis

Sarcoidosis involving the orbit and paranasal sinuses is rare. In one report, there were 2 cases of orbital sarcoid in a series of 1000 cases of orbital tumors.[35] Sarcoid can involve the paranasal sinuses and invade the orbit.[36] Ocular sarcoid can involve almost any part of the eye or its adnexa. Exophthalmos may be the presenting sign.[37] Any part of the optic nerve along the anterior visual pathway can be affected; this includes involvement of the optic chiasm and erosion of the optic canal.[38,39] Optic nerve involvement can take four forms, resulting in papilledema, optic neuritis, optic atrophy, and optic nerve granulomas.

The CT findings are variable. There may be thickening of the scleral margin of the globe, with probable involvement of the adjacent Tenon's capsule. This resembles pseudotumor. A nonspecific soft-tissue density may occupy the retrobulbar area, often extending up to and abutting the globe. Thickening of the optic nerve may also occur.

Mucormycosis (Phycomycosis)

This fungal infection may involve the orbit, sinuses, nose, oral cavity, soft tissues of the face, and the central nervous system. Approximately 50 percent of patients with cerebral mucormycosis have diabetes, the disease is usually poorly controlled, with the patient in acidosis.[40] Immunocompromised patients are also at risk. Mucormycosis should be suspected in any diabetic with ophthalmoplegia, ptosis, proptosis, and neurologic signs of meningoencephalitis. The infection usually originates in the nasal fossa or sinuses and spreads to the orbit.[41] The intracranial cavity can be invaded via the cribriform plate or through the orbital apex.

CT demonstrates the sinus disease with adjacent involvement of the medial orbital structures.[42] The picture is rather similar to that in acute orbital cellulitis. CT findings of sinus disease with focal areas of mucosal thickening and adjacent increased density of the medial orbital fat, with possible swelling of the medial rectus muscle, in a poorly controlled diabetic should arouse suspicions for mucormycosis. Spread into the intracranial cavity can occur rapidly, with CT demonstration of low-absorption areas and abscess formation in the frontal lobes.[43]

Wegener's Granulomatosis

Wegener's granulomatosis is a systemic vasculitis with granulomatous features involving primarily the upper and lower respiratory tracts and kidneys. Ocular manifestations are common, including conjunctivitis, scleritis, and episcleritis, uveitis, and optic neuritis.[44] The membranes of the nose and sinuses break down with extension of this aggressive necrotizing process into the orbit. A pseudotumor-like picture with chronic granulomatous changes is characteristic.[45,46] CT demonstrates the sinus involvement with varying degrees of bone destruction and unilateral or bilateral orbital masses.[47] Orbital involvement without apparent sinus disease may also occur.

REFERENCES

1. Gellady AM, Shulman ST, Ayoub EM: Periorbital and orbital cellulitis in children. Pediatrics 61:272–277, 1978
2. Haynes RE, Cramblett HG: Acute ethmoiditis: its relationship to orbital cellulitis. Am J Dis Child 114:261–267, 1967
3. Jarrett WH, Gutman FA: Ocular complications of infection in the paranasal sinuses. Arch Ophthalmol 81:683–688, 1969
4. Fearon B, Edmonds B, Bird R: Orbital-facial complications of sinusitis in children. Laryngoscope 89:947–952, 1979
5. Batson OV: Relationship of the eye to the paranasal sinuses. Arch Ophthalmol 16:322–328, 1936
6. Wolff E: Anatomy of the Eye and Orbit, 7th ed. Philadelphia, WB Saunders, 1976, pp 191–194
7. Williams PL, Warwick R: Functional Neuroanatomy of Man. Philadelphia, WB Saunders, 1975, p 1130
8. Chandler JR, Langenbrunner DJ, Stevens ER: The pathogenesis of orbital complications in acute sinusitis. Laryngoscope 80:1414–1428, 1970
9. Goldberg F, Berne AS, Oski FA: Differentiation of orbital cellulitis from preseptal cellulitis by computed tomography. Pediatrics 62:1000–1005, 1978
10. Leo JS, Halpern J, Sackler JP: Computed tomography in the evaluation of orbital infections. Comput Tomogr 4:133–138, 1980
11. Zimmerman RA, Bilaniuk LT: CT of orbital infection and its cerebral complications. AJR 134:45–50, 1980
12. Fernbach SK, Naidich TP: CT diagnosis of orbital inflammation in children. Neuroradiology 22:7–13, 1981
13. Harr DL, Quencer RM, Abrams GW: Computed tomography and ultrasound in the evaluation of orbital infection and pseudotumor. Radiology 142:395–401, 1982
14. Jakobiec FA, Jones IS: Orbital Inflammations. In Jones IS, Jakobiec FA (eds): Diseases of the Orbit. Hagerstown, Md., Harper & Row, 1979, pp 187–261
15. Jellinek EH: The orbital pseudotumour syndrome and its differentiation from endocrine exophthalmos. Brain 92:35–58, 1969
16. Blodi FC, Gass JDM: Inflammatory pseudotumor of the orbit. Trans Am Acad Ophthalmol Otolaryngol 71:303–323, 1967
17. Zimmerman LE: Lymphoid tumors. In Boniuk M (ed): Ocular and Adnexal Tumors: New and Controversial Aspects. St. Louis, Mosby, 1964, p 429
18. Jakobiec FA, McLean I, Font RL: Clinicopathologic characteristics of orbital lymphoid hyperplasia. Ophthalmology (Rochester) 86:948–966, 1979
19. Nugent RA, Rootman J, Robertson WD, Lapointe JS, Harrison PB: Acute orbital pseudotumors: classification and CT features. AJR 137:957–962, 1981
20. Enzmann D, Donaldson SS, Marshall WH, Kriss JP: Computed tomography in orbital pseudotumor (idiopathic orbital inflammation). Radiology 120:597–601, 1976
21. Bernardino ME, Zimmerman RD, Citrin CM, Davis DO: Scleral thickening: a CT sign of orbital pseudotumor. AJR 129:703–706, 1977
22. Trokel SL, Hilal SK: Computed tomography of orbital and ocular tumors. In Jakobiec FA (ed): Ocular and Adnexal Tumors. Birmingham, Ala. Aesculapius Publishing, 1978, pp 257–270
23. Dallow RL: Personal communication, 1982
24. Eshaghian J, Anderson RL: Sinus involvement in inflammatory orbital pseudotumor. Arch Ophthalmol 99:627–630, 1981
25. Trokel SL, Hilal SK: Recognition and differential diagnosis of enlarged extraocular muscles in computed tomography. Am J Ophthalmol 87:503–512, 1979
26. Hurwitz BS, Atrin CM: Use of computerized axial tomography (CAT scan) in evaluating therapy of orbital pseudotumors. Ann Ophthalmol 11:217–221, 1979
27. Moss HM: Expanding lesions of the orbit. A clinical study of 230 consecutive cases. Am J Ophthalmol 54:761–770, 1962
28. Youssefi B: Orbital tumors in children. A clinical study of 62 cases. J Pediatr Ophthalmol 6:177–185, 1969
29. Enzmann DR, Donaldson SS, Kriss JP: Appearance of Graves' disease on orbital computed tomography. J Comput Assist Tomogr 3:815–819, 1979

30. Werner SC: Orbital changes in Graves' disease. In Jones IS and Jakobiec FA (eds): Diseases of the Orbit. Hagerstown, Md., Harper & Row, 1979, pp 263–267

31. Cohen BA, Som PM, Haffner PH, Friedman AH: Steroid exophthalmos. J Comput Assist Tomogr 5:907–908, 1981

32. Ossoinig KC: Standardized echography: basic principals, clinical applications, and results. In Dallow RL (ed): Ophthalmic Ultrasonography Comparative Techniques. Boston, Little, Brown, 1979, pp 165–173

33. Brismar J, Davis KR, Dallow RL, Brismar G: Unilateral endocrine exophthalmos. Diagnostic problems in association with computed tomography. Neuroradiology 12:21–24, 1976

34. Healy JF, Metcalf JH, Brahme FJ: Thyroid ophthalmopathy: bony erosion on CT and increased vascularity on angiography. AJNR 2:472–474, 1981

35. Benedict WL: Sarcoidosis involving the orbit. Arch Ophthalmol 42:546–550, 1949

36. Bronson LJ, Fisher YL: Sarcoidosis of the paranasal sinuses with orbital extension. Arch Ophthal 94:243–244, 1976

37. Melmon KL, Goldberg JS; Sarcoidosis with bilateral exophthalmos as the initial symptom. Am J Med 33:158–160, 1962

38. Jampol LM, Woodfin W, McLean EB: Optic nerve sarcoidosis. Arch Ophthalmol 87:355–360, 1972

39. James DG, Zatouroff JT, Rose FC: Papilloedema in sarcoidosis. Br J Ophthalmol 51:526–529, 1967

40. Fleckner RA, Goldstein JH: Mucormycosis. Br J Ophthalmol 53:542–548, 1969

41. Baum JL: Rhino-orbital mucormycosis. Am J Ophthalmol 63:335–339, 1967

42. Centeno RS, Bentson JR, Mancuso AA: CT scanning in rhinocerebral mucormycosis and aspergillosis. Radiology 140:383–389, 1981

43. Lazo A, Wilner HI, Metes JJ: Craniofacial mucormycosis: computed tomographic and angiographic findings in two cases. Radiology 139:623–626, 1981

44. Haynes BF, Fishman ML, Fauci AS, Wolff SM: The ocular manifestations of Wegener's granulomatosis: fifteen years experience and review of the literature. Am J Med 63:131–141, 1977

45. Faulds JS, Wear AR: Pseudotumour of the orbit and Wegener's granuloma. Lancet 2:955–957, 1960

46. Weiter J, Farkas TG: Pseudotumor of the orbit as a presenting sign in Wegener's granulomatosis. Surv Ophthalmol 17:106–119, 1972

47. Vermess M, Haynes BF, Fauci AS, Wolff SM: Computer assisted tomography of orbital lesions in Wegener's granulomatosis. J Comput Assist Tomogr 2:45–48, 1978

48. Green WR, Font RL, Zimmerman LE: Aspergillosis of the orbit. Arch Ophthalmol 82:302–313, 1969

49. Olurin O, Lucas AO, Oyediran ABO: Orbital histoplasmosis due to histoplasma duboisii. Am J Ophthalmol 68:14–18, 1969

50. Vida L, Moel SA: Systemic North American blastomycosis with orbital involvement. Am J Ophthalmol 77:240–242, 1974

51. Streeten B, Rabuzzi DD, Jones DB: Sporotrichosis of the orbital margin. Am J Ophthalmol 77:750–755, 1974

52. Baghdassarian SA, Zakharia H: Hydatid cyst: report of 3 cases. Am J Ophthalmol 71:1081–1084, 1971

53. Talib H: Orbital hydatid disease in Iraq. Br J Surg 59:391–394, 1972

54. Knowles DM, Jakobiec FA, Rosen M, Howard G: Amyloidosis of the orbit and adnexae. Surv Ophthalmol 19:367–384, 1975

55. Raab EL: Intraorbital amyloid. Br J Ophthal 54:445–449, 1970

56. Howard GM: Amyloid tumours of the orbit. Br J Ophthalmol 50:421–425, 1966

57. Mortada A: Tuberculoma of the orbit and lacrimal gland. Br J Ophthalmol 55:565–567, 1971

CASE 1. Periorbital Cellulitis

A 47-year-old female with painful swollen area over left mandible for four days. Swelling spread to face and forehead. Examination revealed diffuse left facial swelling, with erythema extending from mandible to cheek, ear, and forehead. Temperature 103 F. Eye examination normal.

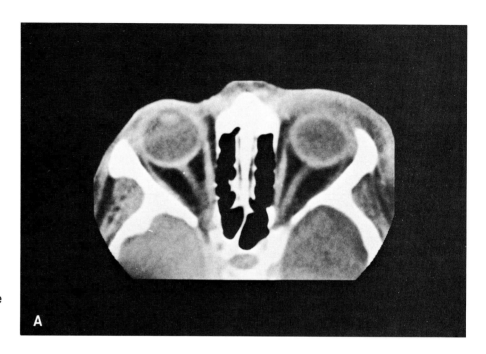

Figure A. Preseptal soft-tissue swelling is present on the left. The ethmoid sinuses and retrobulbar regions are normal.

Diagnosis: Periorbital cellulitis, probably of dental origin.

CASE 2. Post-traumatic Periorbital Cellulitis

This 31-year-old female was assaulted and suffered lacerations above and below the right eye two days prior to admission. Presented with painful, swollen periorbital area. Eye examination very limited due to the considerable swelling of the eyelids.

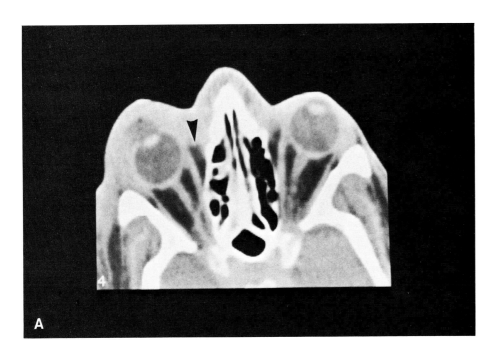

Figure A. Marked preseptal periorbital swelling is present bilaterally, greater on the right. The preseptal area is sharply demarcated at the orbital septum (arrowhead). The retrobulbar areas are normal.

CASE 3. Post-traumatic Periorbital Cellulitis

This five-year-old female sustained a laceration over left eye. Twelve hours later, she developed periorbital swelling and erythema. She was febrile with leucocytosis, and the laceration was purulent. Eye examination was normal. No proptosis.

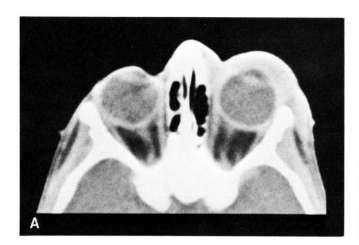 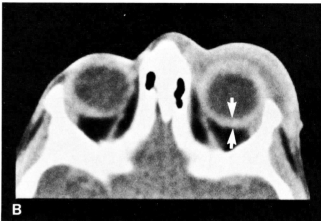

Figures A and B. There is preseptal swelling involving the anterior soft tissues. Note the thickened margin of the entire left globe in B (arrows). This apparent thickening of the scleral margin is probably largely due to an inflammatory effusion in Tenon's space.

Follow-up: The patient was treated with parenteral antibiotics with rapid resolution of the inflammatory process.

CASE 4. Sinusitis with Periorbital Cellulitis

A 14-year-old female with a one-week history of nasal congestion, head-aches, and fever who developed right periorbital swelling. Eye examination normal except for conjunctival injection and chemosis. No proptosis or limita-tion of extraocular muscle motion. There was swelling of the right eyelids, which extended up to the forehead and across the midline. Purulent material was draining into the nasal fossa.

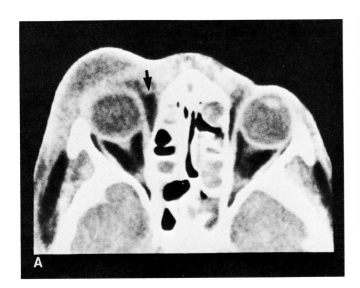

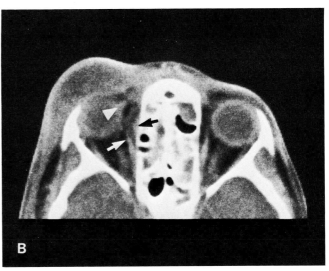

Figure A. Parital opacification of both ethmoid sinuses is present, confirming the diagnosis of ethmoiditis. Right-sided periorbital swelling is present. Note the sharp limitation of the edematous preseptal tissues at the orbital septum (arrow). The medial rectus muscle is intact.

Figure B. CT section slightly craniad to A. At this level, the superior oblique muscle (white arrow) is displaced away from the ethmoid plate by a small subperiosteal abscess (black arrow). Note the insertion of the tendon of the superior oblique muscle into the globe (arrow-head) is posterior to the orbital septum.

Follow-up: Clearing of inflammatory process with parenteral antibiotics.

CASE 5. Periorbital Swelling Due to Non-Hodgkin's Lymphoma
This 59-year-old male noted painless sagging of right upper eyelid. Examination revealed a swollen eyelid with a palpable nodular mass on the lateral aspect of the upper eyelid. There was limitation of lateral gaze.

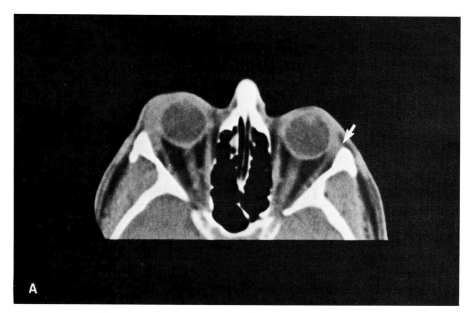

Figure A. There is a soft-tissue mass involving the right lateral periorbital area, extending laterally to involve the lacrimal gland. Compare with the opposite side to identify a normal lacrimal gland (arrow). The CT appearance of the periorbital swelling is identical to that of typical inflammatory disease (compare with Case 13).

Follow-up: Biopsy of the palpebral lobe of the right lacrimal gland revealed non-Hodgkin's lymphoma.

CASE 6. Sinusitis with Orbital Cellulitis and Subperiosteal Abscess

An 11-year-old male with headache and fever for four days, with recent onset of swelling of right eyelid. Examination revealed edematous, erythematous right eyelid. No proptosis. Conjunctiva mildly injected. Fundoscopy normal. Extraocular muscle mobility normal. Sinus opacification demonstrated on routine radiographs. A diagnosis of sinusitis with periorbital cellulitis was made. Following three days of IV antibiotic therapy, the patient developed mild proptosis with limitation of extraocular motion. CT scan was performed at that time.

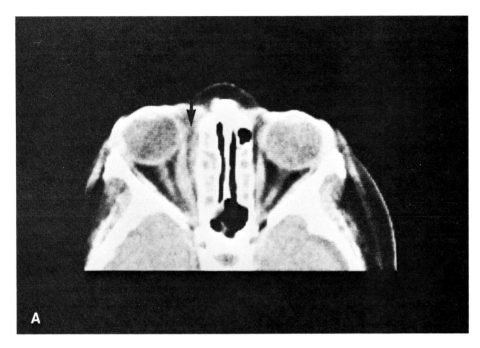

Figure A. Both ethmoid sinuses are opacified. The right medial rectus muscle is markedly swollen. The periorbita is elevated, indicating a subperiosteal abscess. The fat plane between the medial rectus and periorbita has a mottled configuration (arrow), indicating orbital involvement with the inflammatory infiltrate.

Follow-up: By the seventh day of antibiotic therapy considerable improvement had occurred. No surgical drainage procedure was performed.

CASE 7. Sinusitis with Orbital Cellulitis
A 25-year-old male with history of sinusitis and recent onset of painful proptosis on the right.

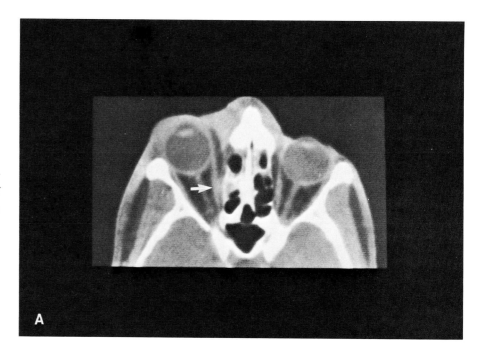

Figure A. There is moderate opacification of the midright ethmoid air cells. Immediately adjacent to this, the periorbita is minimally elevated, suggesting a small subperiosteal collection. The adjacent medial rectus muscle (arrow) is thickened due to swelling from orbital cellulitis. The globe is proptosed forwards. Preseptal swelling is also present.

CASE 8. Sinusitis with Orbital and Periorbital Cellulitis

A 13-year-old male with trauma to forehead. He subsequently developed swelling of the left periorbital area, which became progressively worse over several days. No prior history of sinus disease.

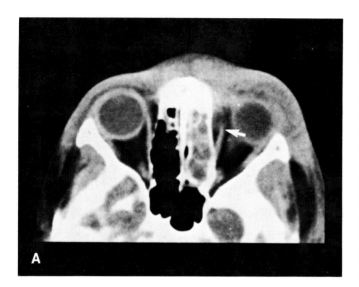

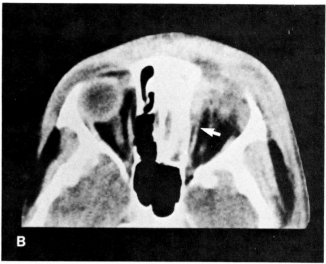

Figure A. There is bilateral periorbital swelling, more marked on the left. The left ethmoid sinus is opacified. The left medial rectus muscle is laterally displaced (arrow) by infiltration of the medial extraconal space.

Figure B. CT section more craniad than in A, demonstrating lateral displacement of the superior oblique muscle (arrow), secondary to the orbital infiltration. The periorbital swelling and left ethmoid opacification are noted.

Follow-up: Patient responded well to parenteral antibiotics.

CASE 9. Sinusitis: Orbital Cellulitis with Subperiosteal Abscess

A 12-year-old male with 3-day history of headache. Awoke at night with right-sided proptosis. Examination revealed swelling, erythema, and tenderness of right eyelid. Hertel exophthalmometer readings: 27 mm OD, 15 mm OS, at 90-mm base. Restricted mobility in all directions on right. Right disc flat with slight venous engorgement. Visual acuity: 20/50 OD, 20/25 OS. Purulent material draining from middle turbinates.

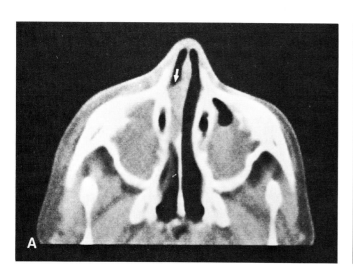

Figure A. Both maxillary antra are opacified, with a small air-fluid level on the left. Partial opacification on the right nasal fossa (arrow) is probably due to draining purulent material. There is facial swelling overlying the right antrum.

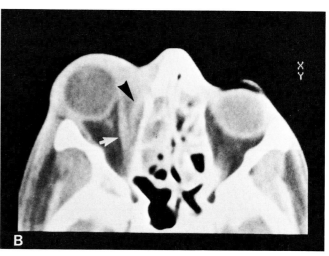

Figure B. Proptosis is present on the right. The medial rectus muscle is thickened (arrow), secondary to the adjacent inflammatory process. This indicates early orbital cellulitis. The periosteum is elevated (arrowhead), indicating a subperiosteal abscess. The ethmoid sinuses are opacified. Preseptal periorbital swelling is also present anteriorly.

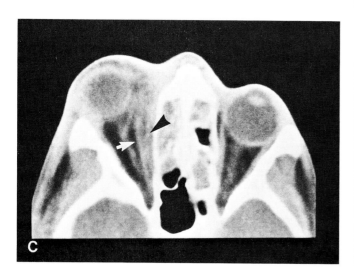

Figure C. At a slightly more craniad level than B, the superior oblique muscle is laterally displaced (arrow) by the elevated periorbita (arrowhead).

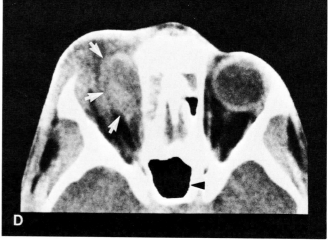

Figure D. CT section through the upper right orbit reveals a discreet mass (arrows), which probably is part of the subperiosteal abscess. Coronal views were not obtained. The sphenoid sinus is clear (arrowhead).

Follow-up: Despite the CT findings indicating a subperiosteal abscess, the patient responded rapidly to parenteral antibiotics, with complete regression of the proptosis in one week. Surgical drainage was not performed.

CASE 10. Sinusitis with Orbital Cellulitis

This 11-year-old male who had a long history of sinusitis developed rapid onset of orbital pain and swelling. Obvious proptosis was noted on examination. There was limitation of extraocular muscle motion in all directions.

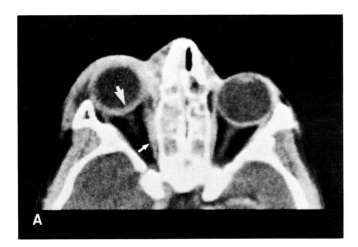

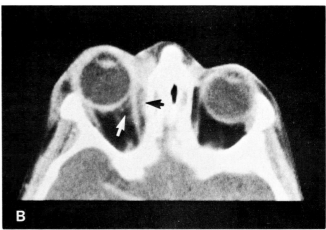

Figure A. Opacification of both ethmoid sinuses is present, confirming the ethmoiditis. Right-sided proptosis is noted. The right medial rectus muscle is thickened (small arrow), indicating inflammatory involvement. Right periorbital swelling is noted anteriorly. The margin of the globe is uniformly thickened (large arrow), suggesting inflammatory effusion of Tenon's space. Note the difference in the configuration of the retrobulbar fat between the two sides. On the involved right side, there is an overall increase in density with a stippled configuration, compared to the uniform black orbital fat on the normal left side. This indicates infiltration of the intraconal retrobulbar fat with the inflammatory process.

Follow-up: Resolution with antibiotic therapy.

Figure B. CT section slightly craniad to A. Again note the stippled appearance of the intraconal retrobulbar fat (white arrow). There is a minimal periosteal reaction medially (black arrow).

CASE 11. Sinusitis with Orbital Cellulitis

A 42-year-old male with chronic sinusitis presented with recent onset of painful left orbital swelling. Examination revealed left periorbital swelling, proptosis, chemosis, and limitation of extraocular motion.

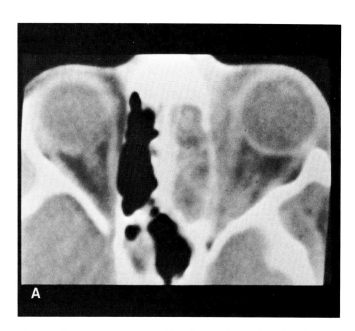

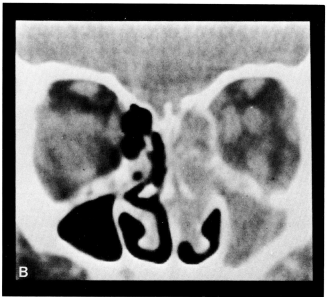

Figure A. Complete opacification of left ethmoid sinus is noted. There is increased density involving the entire retrobulbar fat pad, indicating spread of the inflammatory infiltrate. The medial rectus muscle is swollen. The eye is proptotic.

Figure B. Coronal CT demonstrates opacification of the left maxillary antrum, ethmoid sinus, and upper nasal fossa. Infiltration of the left retrobulbar area is manifest by multiple stippled densities. The medial rectus muscle is thickened and laterally displaced. The large central density occupying the right orbit is the normal posterior globe, surrounded by normal-appearing orbital fat.

Follow-up: The patient underwent a sinus drainage procedure with eventual resolution of the inflammatory process.

CASE 12. Acute Dacryoadenitis

A 42-year-old female presented with left orbital pain aggravated by eye movements. Examination revealed erythematous, swollen lid and conjuctiva injected with chemosis. A tender mass was palpated in the superolateral quadrant.

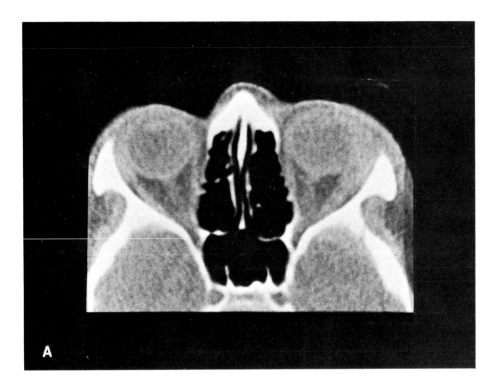

Figure A. A soft-tissue mass is present lateral to the globe, with adjacent anterior swelling. A soft-tissue mass extends posteriorly, with swelling of the lacteral rectus muscle.*

Follow-up: Resolution with antibiotic therapy.

*Reprinted from Hesselink JR, Davis KR, Dallow RL, et al: Computed tomography of masses in the lacrimal gland region. Radiology 131:146, 1979, with permission.

CASE 13. Periorbital Cellulitis and Dacryoadenitis
A 10-year-old male with progressive left eyelid swelling for 3 days. Treated with antihistamines and steroids without improvement.

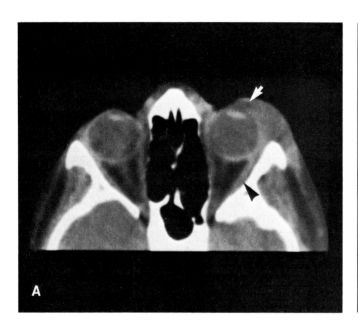

Figure A. The anterior soft-tissue swelling extends into the lateral aspect of the orbit and posteriorly with swelling of the lateral rectus muscle (arrowhead). The small lucency (arrow) represents air trapped in the palpebral fissure.

Figure B. Coronal CT demonstrating soft-tissue swelling in the superolateral quadrant of the orbit encompassing the region of the lacrimal gland fossa.

Follow-up: Resolution of inflammatory process with parenteral antibiotics.

CASE 14. Sinusitis with Subperiosteal Abscess

A 12-year-old female with fever, headache, and left periorbital swelling. Examination revealed marked left proptosis and limitation of extraocular motion. Conjuctiva injected with chemosis. Visual acuity was decreased.

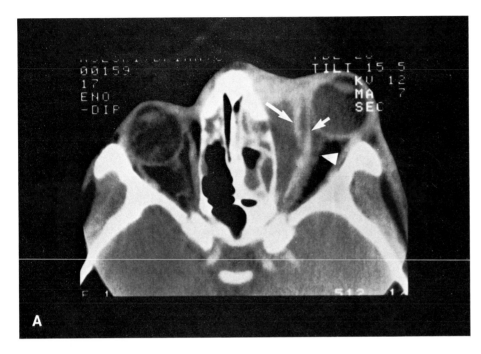

Figure A. Left ethmoid opacification is present. There is a large homogeneous density occupying the medial left orbital area. This represents the subperiosteal abscess, which has displaced the periosteum (large arrow) laterally. The periosteum has enhanced with contrast. The periosteum abuts the displaced medial rectus muscle (small arrow). The optic nerve is stretched (arrowhead).

Follow-up: The subperiosteal abscess was surgically drained.

CASE 15. Sinusitis, Orbital Cellulitis, and Subperiosteal Abscess
This 11-year-old male had a 4-day history of headache, left eye pain, and swelling, with inability to open eyelid. Temperature, 104 F. Proptosis of 10 mm OS; total ophthalmoplegia. Pupil and fundus normal. Visual acuity: 20/50 OS, 20/20 OD. Sinus radiographs revealed pansinusitis.

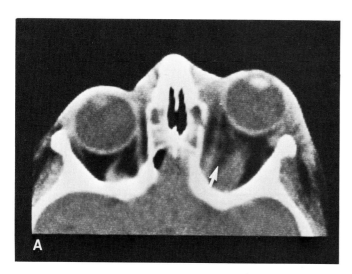

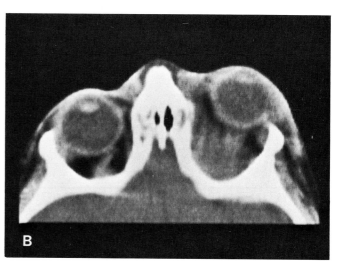

Figure A. Initial CT performed soon after admission demonstrates bilateral ethmoid opacification, marked proptosis, and anterior periorbital swelling. There is increased density involving the retrobulbar fat (arrow), which is present between the superior rectus and medial rectus muscles. This indictes the presence of retrobulbar infiltrate, confirming the diagnosis of orbital cellulitis.

Figure B. Slightly more craniad, this section demonstrates a diffuse abnormal density in the upper orbit. A coronal view would be necessary for precise localization.

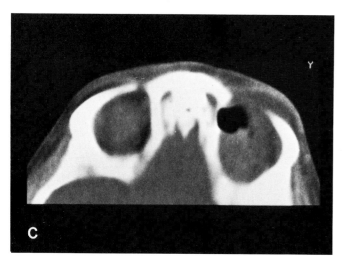

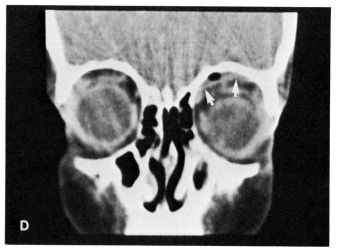

Figure C. After 10 days of antibiotic therapy, there was some initial improvement, but progress had plateaued. Repeat axial CT reveals air in the upper orbit.

Figure D. Coronal CT demonstrates some clearing of the sinuses, although residual sinus opacification was present at other levels. The air occupies a subperiosteal abscess cavity. Note the superior periosteum, which has been depressed by the subperiosteal abscess (arrows). This subperiosteal abscess corresponds to the superior orbital density on the previous CT in B, 10 days earlier.

Follow-up: At this stage the patient underwent bilateral maxillary sinus drainage and a left intranasal ethmoidectomy. He was discharged after three weeks of hospitalization with residual mild proptosis.

CASE 16. Sinusitis and Orbital Abscess
Following underwater diving, this 15-year-old male developed headache, nausea, and rapid progressive left orbital swelling. Examination revealed marked left proptosis, limitation of extraocular motion, chemosis, and retinal hemorrhage with only light perception.

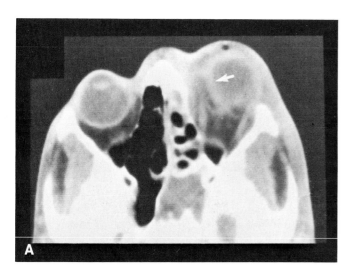

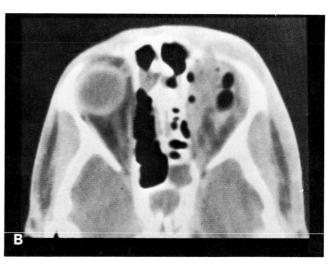

Figure A. Marked left proptosis and periorbital swelling are present. The rim of the globe is thickened (arrow), suggesting a Tenon's capsule effusion. There is increased density of the retrobulbar fat delineating the orbital infiltrate. The left ethmoid sinus is partially opacified. The left sphenoid sinus is completely dense.

Figure B. CT section slightly craniad to A demonstrates a diffuse increase in retrobulbar density with air bubbles.

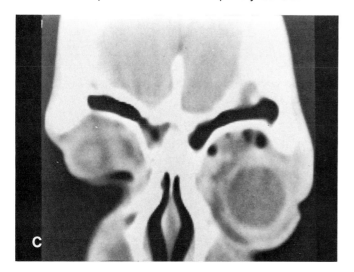

Figure C. Coronal CT demonstrates diffuse increase in density of the periocular orbital fat with air bubbles, confirming the diagnosis of orbital abscess.

Follow-up: The patient underwent a left external ethmoidectomy, sphenoidotomy, and drainage of a periorbital and orbital abscess.

CASE 17. Acute Orbital Pseudotumor

A 55-year-old female with one-day history of itchy, swollen left eye. Examination revealed left proptosis, chemosis, and erythematous, indurated, edematous eyelids. There was reduced globe motility with increased orbital resistance. The pupil, fundus, and vision were normal.

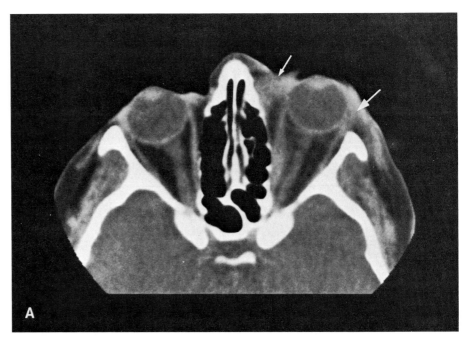

Figure A. Left exophthalmos is present. Discreet soft-tissue densities are present in the medial canthal area (small arrow) and around the lacrimal gland (large arrow). The medial rectus muscle is thickened. There is increased density of the retrobulbar fat.

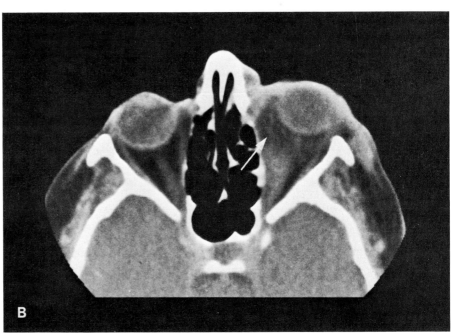

Figure B. Section more craniad than A demonstrates the diffuse mottling of the retrobulbar fat (arrow), indicating involvement with the inflammatory infiltrate. Compare with the normal retrobulbar fat on the right side.

Follow-up: There was a dramatic response to steroid therapy, with resolution within two days.

CASE 18. Pseudotumor: Reactive Lymphoid Hyperplasia
This 29-year-old male had a history of recurrent peripheral uveitis OU for several years. Recently, he noted a red mass on the lateral aspect of the eye. No pain or visual symptoms or diplopia. Examination revealed normal vision. Minimal left proptosis with increased resistance to retropulsion.

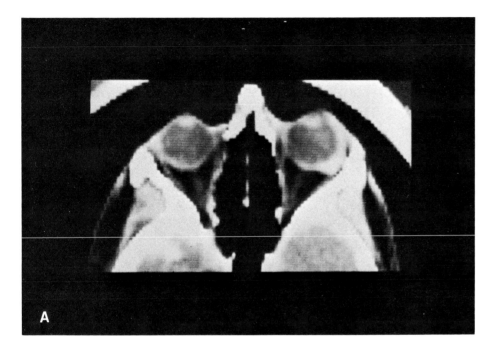

A

Figure A. There is a crescentic-shaped mass around the lateral apsect of the globe that enhanced with contrast.

Follow-up: The mass was excised. Pathologic examination revealed reactive lymphoid hyperplasia. No long-term follow-up available. (Compare with Cases 25–27, and 38.)

CASE 19. Pseudotumor: Benign Lymphoid Hyperplasia

A 62-year-old female with 1-month history of progressive swelling of right upper lid with excessive tearing. A hard, slightly tender mass was palpated in the region of the lacrimal gland. Vision was 20/20 OS, 20/60 OD. Limitation of upgaze on the right.

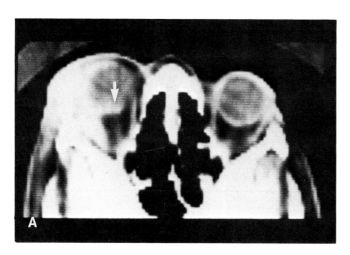

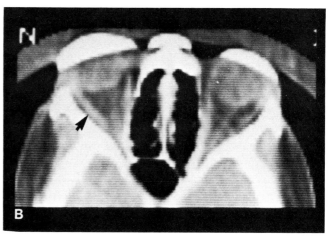

Figure A. CT with contrast reveals an enhancing soft-tissue mass in the region of the lacrimal gland, extending posteriorly to the orbital apex in the lateral extraconal space. The ocular rim is thickened (arrow) and also enhances. The biopsy specimen revealed benign lymphoid hyperplasia.

Figure B. Follow-up scan one year later, after steroid therapy. There has been complete resolution of the soft-tissue mass. Minimal residual thickening of the lateral rectus muscle is present (arrow).

CASE 20. Pseudotumor

A 69-year-old female with 5-month history of puffy left lower eyelid and decreasing vision. Examination revealed left proptosis and edema of the lower lid. Visual acuity: 20/100 OS, 20/40 OD.

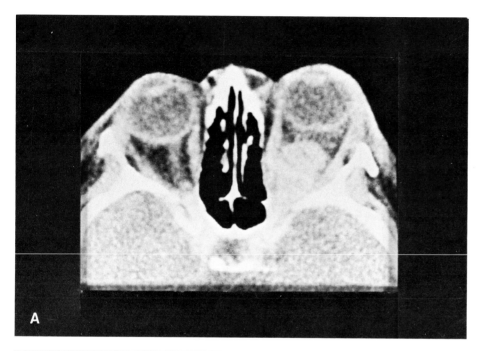

Figure A. Initial CT reveals a well-defined retrobulbar and apical mass. The patient refused biopsy and was treated empirically with steroids.

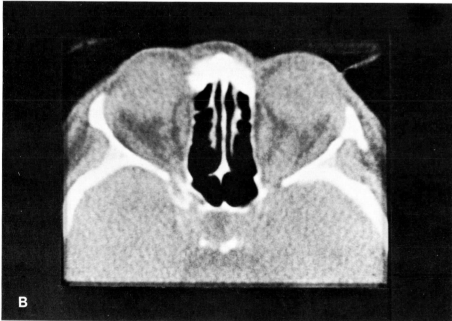

Figure B. Follow-up CT $3\frac{1}{2}$ months later reveals considerable reduction in the size of the mass. There had also been interval visual improvement.

Diagnosis: Presumed pseudotumor, without long-term follow-up.

CASE 21. Pseudotumor: Benign Lymphoid Hyperplasia
A 64-year-old male with progressive right proptosis for several years. Increasing blurred vision on the right. No orbital pain.

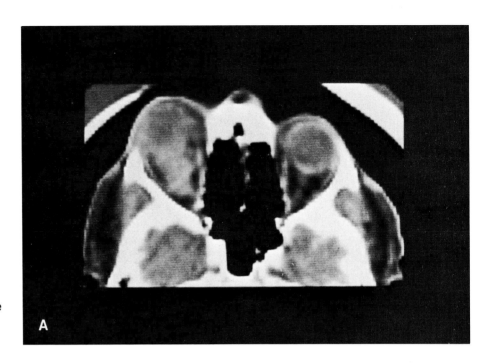

Figure A. There is proptosis on the right with a well-defined lobulated intraconal mass, inseparable from the optic nerve, and abutting the globe.

Follow-up: Posterior orbital exploration with subtotal excision of the mass was performed. Histologic examination revealed benign lymphoid hyperplasia. The patient was referred for radiation therapy.

CASE 22. Sclerosing Pseudotumor

A 23-year-old female with a 5-year history of right sclerosing pseudotumor diagnosed by biopsy via a Kronlein lateral orbitotomy. Treatment with steroids had resulted in some clinical improvement, but the patient remained on a maintenance dose. Vision was normal OU; proptosis of 5 mm OD. Increased orbital resistance with a palpable irregular solid fixed mass along the superotemporal quadrant of the inner orbital rim was present. Ocular motility was full with no diplopia. Fundi were normal.

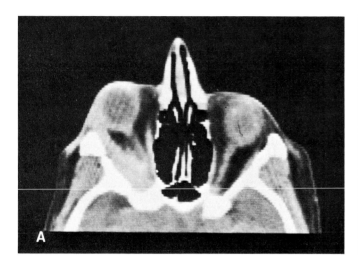 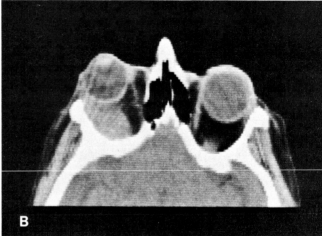

Figures A and B. Axial CTs reveal sharply defined soft-tissue mass encompassing the lacrimal gland fossa and extending posteriorly in the extraconal space to the orbital apex. The mass encroaches on the globe.

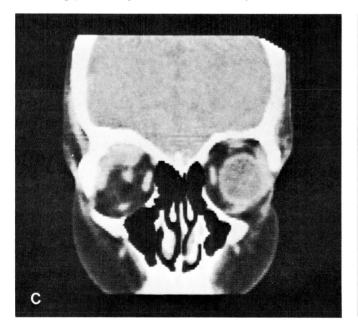 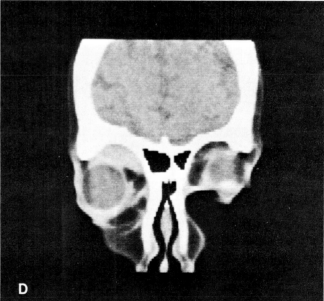

Figures C and D. Coronal CTs demonstrate the soft-tissue mass occupying the superotemporal quadrants. The superior and lateral rectus muscles are contiguous with and inseparable from the mass, as is the lacrimal gland. The mass abuts the globe superiorly.

CASE 23. Pseudotumor: Myositis

A 50-year-old male with prominent left eye for two months. Examination revealed 3 mm of proptosis on left with reduced orbital resilience. Visual acuity: 20/20 OU. Thyroid function tests were normal.

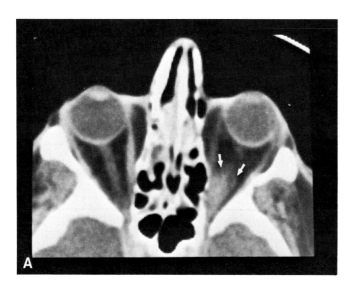

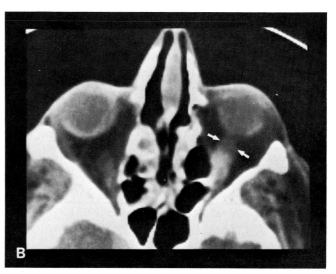

Figure A. An apparent retrobulbar mass extending into the orbital apex is identified (arrows). Ethmoid sinus mucosal thickening is present.

Figure B. Section caudad to A demonstrates asymmetry between the inferior rectus muscles on either side, with enlargement of the left (arrows).

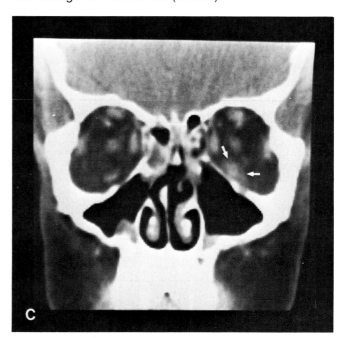

Figure C. Coronal CT confirms the enlarged left inferior rectus muscle (arrows). All the other extraocular muscles are normal. There is mucosal thickening involving both ethmoid and maxillary sinuses.

Follow-up: There was a prompt response to steroid therapy.

CASE 24. Pseudotumor: Myositis

This 28-year-old female developed pain and swelling of right eye 4 weeks after an upper respiratory infection. Examination revealed slight right proptosis and marked limitation of extraocular motion without increased orbital resistance. Vision was normal.

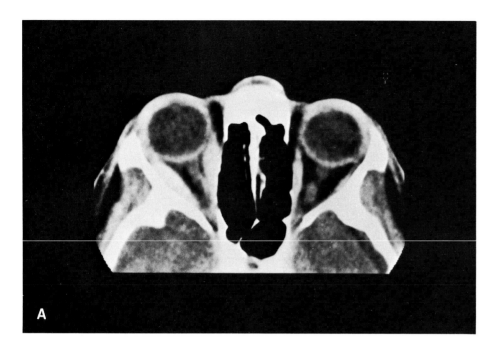

Figure A. The right eye is proptosed forwards. There is considerable thickening of both the medial and lateral rectus muscles, which enhance with contrast.

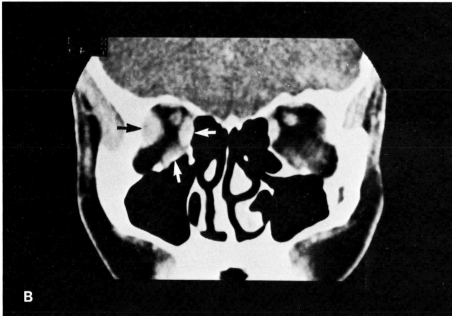

Figure B. Coronal CT reveals thickening of the right lateral rectus (black arrow), medial rectus (medial white arrow), and inferior rectus muscles (inferior white arrow). There is also mild enlargement of the left medial and inferior rectus muscles.

Follow-up: While the patient was undergoing a workup, she spontaneously began to improve. Eventually, she recovered fully without any therapy.

CASE 25. Lymphoma
A 61-year-old woman with disseminated non-Hodgkin's lymphoma presented with slow onset of painless left proptosis. Examination revealed left proptosis, indurated periorbital swelling, and limitation of extraocular motion. Visual acuity was decreased.

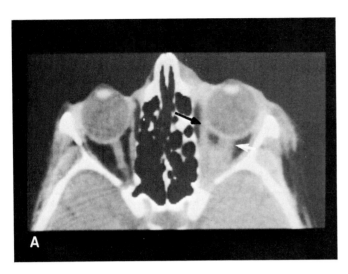

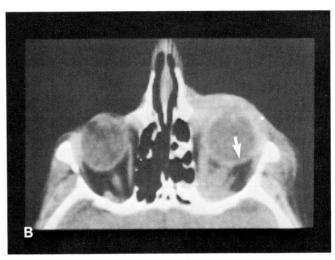

Figure A. A soft-tissue density occupies the orbital apex. The optic nerve (white arrow) and the medial rectus muscle (black arrow) are thickened, probably due to infiltration with lymphoma.

Figure B. Periorbital swelling is noted, indicating involvement of the eyelids. There is thickening of the margin of the globe (arrow), indicating probable infiltration of Tenon's capsule with lymphoma. Note that the retrobulbar fat has increased density compared to the normal right orbit. This suggests infiltration of the fat body.

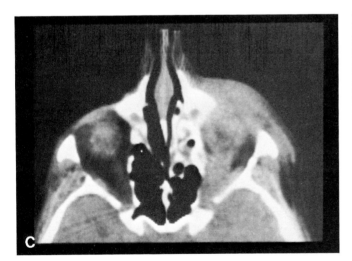

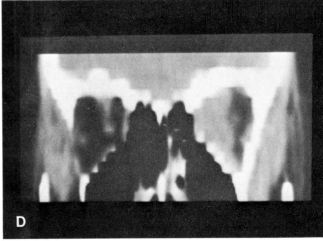

Figure C. CT section through the inferior orbit demonstrates infiltration of lymphoma with involvement of the inferior rectus muscle.

Figure D. Coronal reformatted view demonstrates tumor occupying the medial half of the orbital apex.

CASE 26. Lymphoma
A 67-year-old male with epibulbar lesion on left for 3 months. No change in vision or proptosis.

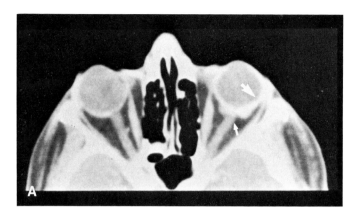

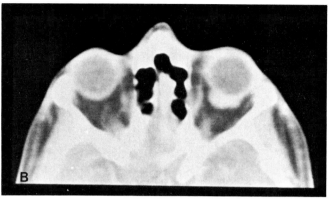

Figure A. There is a discreet soft-tissue mass in the left retrobulbar area abutting the posterior globe. The adjacent margin of the globe is thickened, indicating infiltration of Tenon's capsule (large arrow). Note that the medial rectus muscle appears thickened compared to the medial rectus muscle on the right. However, this does not represent infiltration of the muscle, but is due to unilateral medial rectus contraction secondary to convergent gaze of the left globe. This is determined by the configuration of the optic nerve, which has deviated laterally (small arrow), as the globe rotates.

Figure B. Section craniad to A again demonstrates the discreet well-defined mass adjacent to the posterior globe.

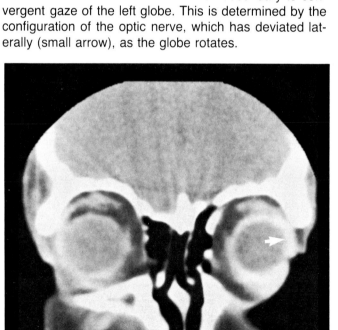

Figure C. Coronal CT reveals thickening of the globe margin (arrow) with a localized soft-tissue mass inferiorly.

Follow-up: Biopsy revealed lymphoma. No systemic lymphoma could be documented.

CASE 27. Lymphoma

A 78-year-old female with left ptosis for a year. Examination revealed non-tender indurated eyelids. Extraocular motion and vision were normal.

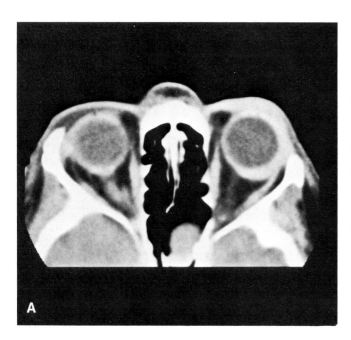 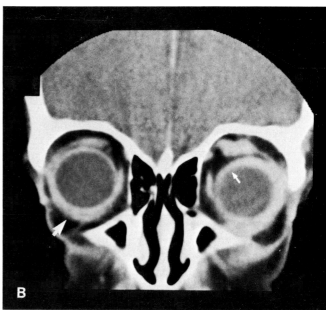

Figures A and B. A well-defined soft-tissue mass surrounds the lateral half of the left globe, involving both anterior and retrobulbar spaces. The rim of the globe is thickened (small arrow), indicating involvement of Tenon's capsule. There is also involvement on the right side (large arrow).

Follow-up: Biopsy revealed lymphoma.

CASE 28. Graves' Disease
A 52-year-old female who had mild clinical hyperthyroidism, including lid retraction. There was no exophthalmos on exophthalmometry. Extrocular motion was full.

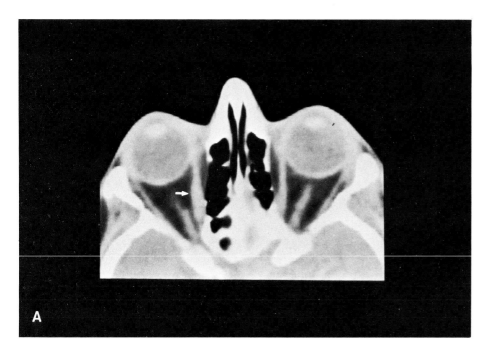

A

Figure A. There is thickening of the right medial rectus muscle (arrow) without involvement of any other extraocular muscles.

CASE 29. Graves' Disease

A 72-year-old male with 6-month history of progressive bilateral orbital swelling and visual deterioration. Examination revealed visual acuity of bare light perception OU. Extraocular movements were limited bilaterally. Hertel measurements were 23 mm OD and 24 mm OS at base 100 mm. Orbital resilience was decreased. Lid edema was present and both upper lids were ptotic.

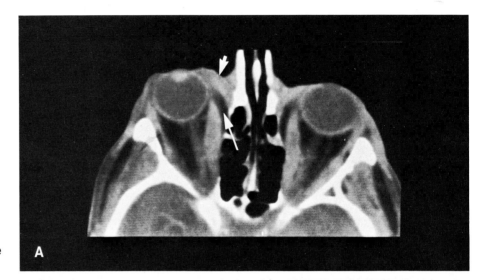

Figure A. The characteristic findings of Graves' disease are present. There is symmetrical thickening of the rectus muscles bilaterally and the orbital fat content is increased (long arrow). In addition, the periorbital soft tissues are thickened (short arrow).

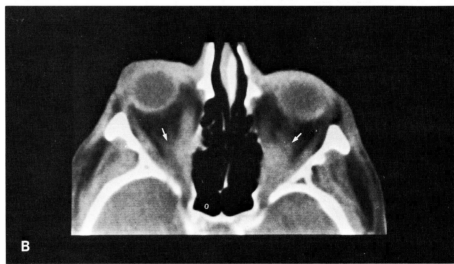

Figure B. Section slightly caudad to A reveals ill-defined densities (arrows) that extend into the apices. These are due to the enlarged inferior rectus muscles.

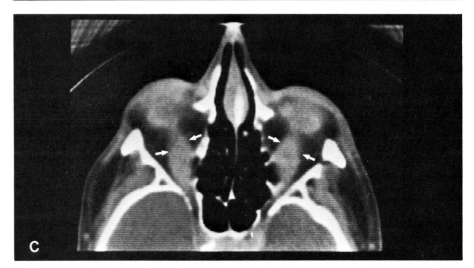

Figure C. Section caudad to B through the lower orbit. Both inferior rectus muscles are identified (arrows) and appear prominent.

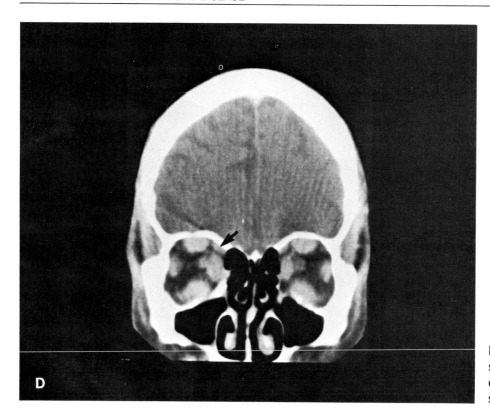

Figure D. Coronal CT confirms symmetrical enlargement of all the extraocular muscles, including the superior oblique muscles (arrow).

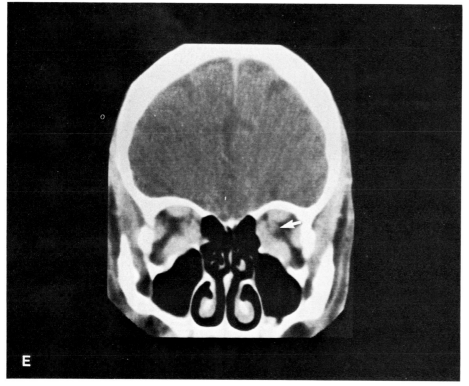

Figure E. Coronal CT posterior to D. Encroachment of the enlarged muscles on the optic nerve (arrow) is apparent. Posterior to this level, the optic nerve could not be separated from the densities of the muscles in the orbital apex, suggesting compression of the nerve bilaterally.

CASE 30. Graves' Disease

This 58-year-old male had a long history of Graves' disease, with continual left orbital inflammation and diplopia.

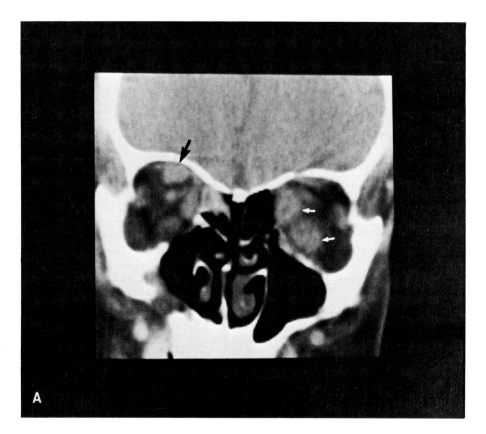

Figure A. Coronal CTs demonstrating asymmetrical enlargement of the extraocular muscles. The medial and inferior rectus muscles (white arrows) in the left orbit are considerably larger than the corresponding muscles on the right. The right superior rectus muscle (black arrow) is much larger than the left.

Follow-up: The patient was referred for strabissmus surgery.

CASE 31. Graves' Disease
This 49-year-old male developed left proptosis and diplopia. Thyroid tests
were positive.

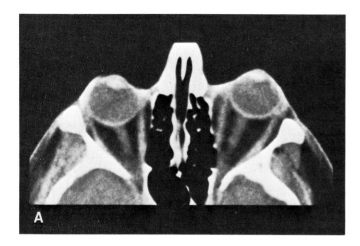

Figure A. The medial and lateral rectus muscles are bilaterally normal. Mild left proptosis is apparent.

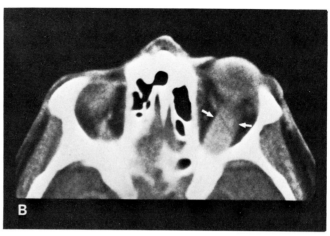

Figure B. CT section craniad to A demonstrates isolated enlargement of the left superior rectus muscle (arrows), accounting for the proptosis.

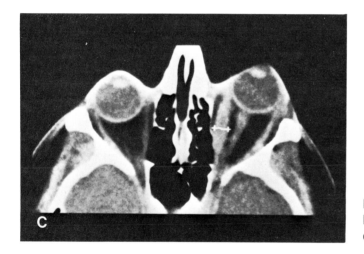

Figure C. Follow-up scan six months later reveals enlargement of the left medial rectus muscle (cursor). The exophthalmos has increased.

CASE 32. Graves' Disease
A 53-year-old female with longstanding history of Graves' disease.

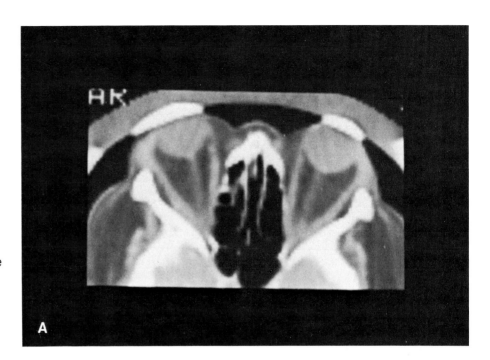

Figure A. The extraocular muscles are prominent, particularly the lateral rectus muscles in both orbits. Of note in this case is the large amount of orbital fat, which is the predominating factor in the causation of the exophthalmos.

CASE 33. Graves' Disease: Status Post-bilateral Ethmoid Lamina Decompression

A 55-year-old female with longstanding Graves' disease. Complete loss of vision OS; OD finger counting only. Bilateral optic atrophy.

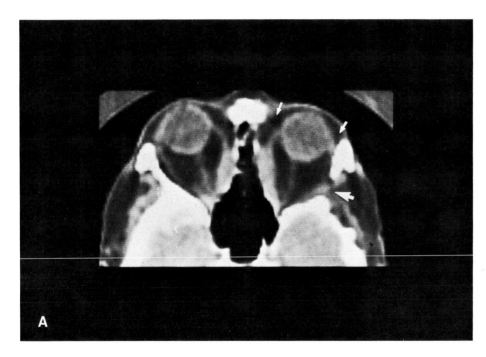

Figure A. Both medial rectus muscles are markedly thickened. There is considerable excess orbital fat anteriorly (small arrows) in both orbits. The ethmoid labyrinth is deformed bilaterally, following the bilateral ethmoid lamina decompressions performed to increase the orbital space. In addition, there is evidence of a previous left Kronlein lateral orbitotomy (large arrow).

CASE 34. Graves' Disease
A 36-year-old male with thyroid disease. Left exophthalmos for a year.

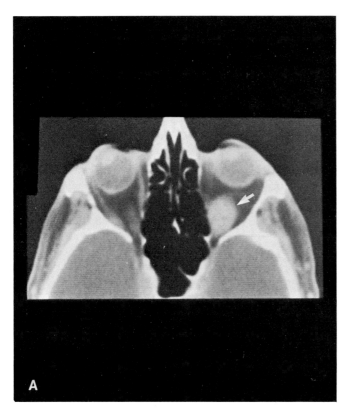

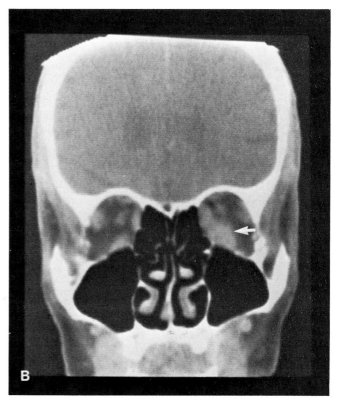

Figure A. An apparent apical density is present on the left.

Figure B. Coronal CT delineates the extraocular muscles to better effect. The apical density seen in A is an enlarged inferior rectus muscle (arrow). In addition, the medial rectus muscle is enlarged.

CASE 35. Graves' Disease
A 57-year old female with history of hyperthyroidism for 15 years treated with radioactive iodine. Thyroid test now normal. Diplopia and progressive right exophthalmos for a year.

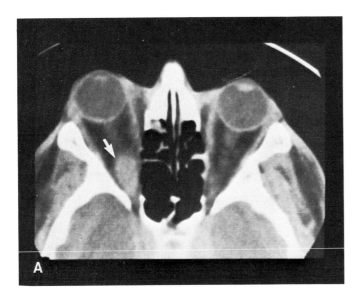 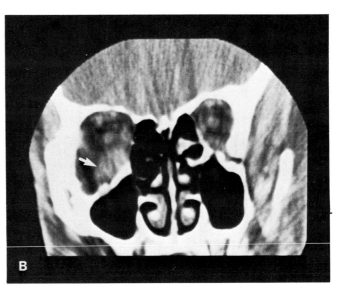

Figure A. Right proptosis is noted. The right medial and lateral rectus muscles appear normal. An apparent apical density is noted (arrow).

Figure B. Coronal CT confirms that the apical density in A is an enlarged inferior rectus muscle (arrow). The linear artifacts in this scan are from dental fillings.

CASE 36. Graves' Disease
A 59-year-old hyperthyroid male with eyelid swelling and decreased vision for two weeks, and intermittent diplopia. Marcus Gunn pupil OD. Visual acuity: 20/60 OS, 20/100 OD. The right optic disc was hyperemic with retinal striae. Extraocular movements were restricted in all directions.

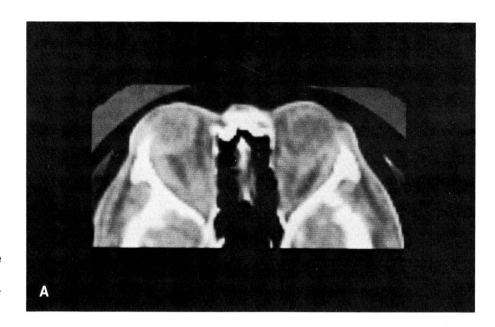

Figure A. The extraocular muscles are bilaterally thickened. In addition, both optic nerves are thickened, more prominent on the right, indicating optic nerve involvement with the thyroid opthalmopathy.

Follow-up: The patient was placed on steroids with considerable improvement in visual acuity.

CASE 37. Sarcoidosis

A 51-year-old black female who presented 6 years earlier with left orbital pain and diplopia but without proptosis. No systemic disease was documented. A retrobulbar mass was identified on ultrasound examination. Biopsy revealed fibrous tissue and chronic inflammatory infiltrate. The patient was treated with steroids for the past 6 years. Recently, she complained of increasing eye pain with lower doses of steroids. Examination revealed 4 mm of exophthalmos. An inflammatory retinal lesion was identified.

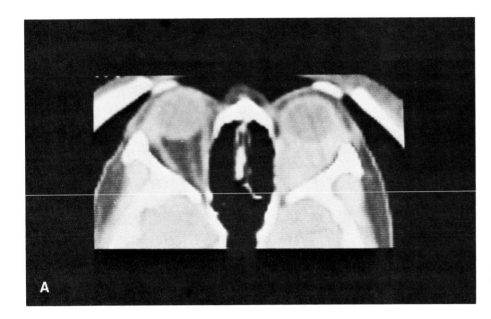

Figure A. There is a diffuse homogeneous mass occupying the entire retrobulbar area, abutting the globe. There was no enhancement with contrast.

Follow-up: A subtotal excision was achieved via a posterior orbital exploration. Histologic examination revealed noncaseating granulomatous infiltrate consistent with sarcoid.

CASE 38. Sarcoidosis

A 30-year-old female with recent onset of blurriness of both eyes. A lung biopsy six months earlier revealed sarcoid. Treated with steroids. Examination on her current admission revealed evidence of a uveitis.

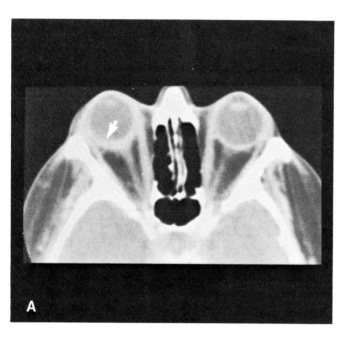

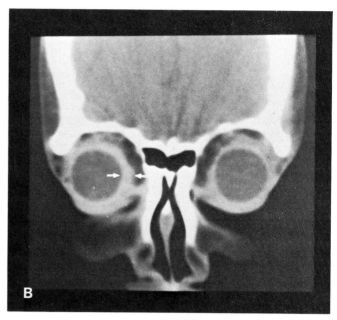

Figure A. The periocular rim of the right globe is thickened (arrow).

Figure B. Coronal CT reveals soft-tissue thickening around both globes, more prominent on the right (arrows). This case reveals similar CT appearances to pseudotumors and lymphoma.

CASE 39. Mucormycosis

A 66-year-old female with a long history of untreated adult-onset diabetes.
Admitted in severe diabetic ketoacidosis and opthalmoplegia for two days.
Examination revealed complete third, fourth, and sixth cranial nerve ophthal-
moplegia OS, with decreased vision. The right eye and orbit were normal.
Lumbar puncture revealed evidence of meningitis.

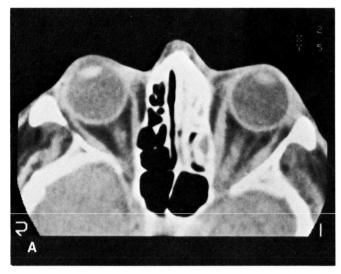

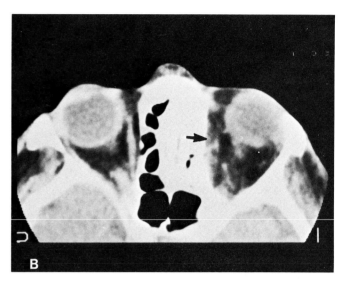

Figure A. There is opacification of the left ethmoid sinus. The septae appear thickened. The left retrobulbar
fat demonstrates a mild diffuse increase in density, indicating involvement with inflammatory infiltrate. The medial and lateral extraocular muscles are thickened, secondary to the inflammatory changes.

Figure B. Section craniad to A reveals a more pro-
nounced orbital density that obliterates the medial extraconal fat (arrow); this is the result of inflammatory
involvement from the adjacent diseased ethmoid sinus.

Follow-up: Mucormycosis was identified from a sinus tap. She subsequently underwent more radical surgery with
appropriate antifungal therapy. The patient subsequently died.

CHAPTER EIGHT

Ocular Lesions

The American Cancer Society anticipates that there will be 1800 new cases of primary malignant tumors of the eye in the next year. These are equally distributed in males and females and will result in 400 deaths.[1] Malignant melanoma of the choroid is the most common primary intraocular tumor, comprising about 75 percent of these lesions, followed by retinoblastoma (20 percent). Epithelial, mesenchymal, and hematopoetic tumors of the uvea, together with meningioma of the optic nerve, comprise the remaining 5 percent.[2]

MALIGNANT MELANOMA *(Cases 1–5)*

Malignant melanomas are rare in children; they appear in all adult age groups, but are most common in the sixth and seventh decades of life. These tumors are almost always single and uniocular, are rare in blacks, and have no gender preference.[3] Familial occurrence of intraocular melanoma is rare.

Malignant melanoma is an invasive neoplasm consisting of cells producing a variable amount of pigment with a potential to spread locally or via blood-borne metastases. The majority appear to arise from preexisting nevi and are most commonly located in the choroid. Melanomas are classified into different cell types: (1) spindle A, (2) spindle B, (3) epithelioid, and (4) mixed (most commonly composed of spindle B and epithelioid). The prognosis of melanoma is influenced adversely when the following parameters are present[2]:

1. larger tumor size
2. predominantly epithelioid cell type
3. heavy pigmentation
4. presence of mytotic activity
5. angle infiltration
6. optic nerve infiltration
7. scleral infiltration
8. extrascleral extension
9. ciliary body infiltration
10. posterior location

Three lesions need to be differentiated from malignant melanoma: metastatic carcinoma,[4] hemangioma, and subretinal hemorrhage.[5-7] In the past, choroidal melanomas were often diagnosed with the ophthalmoscope alone, and errors in diagnosis were frequent. The widespread use of indirect ophthalmoscopy combined with other tests such as fluoroscein angiography, ultrasonography, and the P32 test have increased the rate of early diagnosis and diagnostic accuracy. Correct diagnosis utilizing these modalities can be made in up to 98 percent of cases. With the introduction of high-resolution CT scanners, significant contributions in the diagnosis and extent of eye tumors can be expected,[8] particularly in the determination of extraocular spread.

Malignant melanoma has no characteristic absorption coefficient or enhancement pattern following infusion of contrast material. In the early stages of development, they are characterized by variable thickness of the sclera-uveal layer. If the melanoma spreads widely along the choroid, thickening of the rim of the ocular bulb will be noted. If the lesion extends into the vitreous, a well-defined polypoid mass will be apparent. In large lesions, the entire globe may be involved by the tumor. Extrascleral extension into the orbit and the optic nerve are well defined by CT. In large tumors with invasive characteristics, the lesion may be irregular and fill the entire orbit.[9]

RETINOBLASTOMA (Cases 6–14)

Retinoblastoma is the most common intraocular malignant tumor of childhood, with an incidence varying from 1/17,000 to 1/34,000 live births.[10] The disease usually presents during the first two years of life, although cases have been reported in adults.[11] It may be inherited as an autosomal dominant characterized by a high penetrance. The familial incidence is approximately 10 percent. The vast majority of cases, however, result from sporadic mutations.

Retinoblastoma is rarely diagnosed at an early age unless a family history leads to early evaluation of the eye.[12] The most common finding is leukocoria, which is a white pupillary reflex. Other findings are strabismus and a painful, red eye with or without glaucoma. Other less common findings are nystagmus, hyphema, uveitis, heterochromia iridis, mydriasis and orbital cellulitis. Exophthalmos is less common and occurs only when the tumor has extended into the orbit.

About 34 percent of patients have multiple, independent foci of tumor within the eye. Tumors in the contralateral eye are encountered in about 30 percent of cases. A child with bilateral lesions has a 50 percent chance of passing the disease to his offspring, whereas a child with a sporadic, unilateral retinoblastoma has a 10 to 15 percent chance of doing so. Children with bilateral and hereditary retinoblastomas are particularly susceptible to radiation-induced tumors. They also have a high incidence of second nonocular tumors, often sarcomas, remote from the orbit, which can manifest years after they have survived the bilateral retinoblastomas.

The tumor spreads by implantation that may involve any site within the eye such as the choroidal surface, retinal surface and posterior corneal surface, or the region of the angle. The most commonly encountered varieties are the endophytic and exophytic types. In the more common endophytic type, the tumor arises from the internal nuclear layer of the retina and extends into the vitreous. In the exophytic type, the tumor arises in the external nuclear layers and grows into the subretinal space, causing retinal detachment. The most frequent form of extraocular extension is along the optic nerve, which has been reported in 12.7 percent of cases.[13] If the tumor penetrates the rim of the eye, orbital involvement is encountered; this occurred in 8 percent of one reported series.[14] Hematogenous metastases may be found in the bone marrow, liver, and lung.

CT has contributed significantly to the diagnosis of retinoblastoma and is most valuable in the assessment of tumor extension beyond the globe.[15–17] One finds well-defined, high-density areas arising from the retina. Calcifications are demonstrated within the tumor in high percentages. Small lesions reveal a well-defined tumor margin. In large lesions, the tumor is irregular and the globe is enlarged. Extrascleral spread is reflected by variable-sized tumor masses within the orbit. Optic nerve extension is characterized by thickening of the optic nerve. The optic canal may be enlarged. If the tumor enters the subarachnoid space of the optic nerve, intracranial extension may occur. This is indicated by tumor masses in the suprasellar cistern of the intracranial cavity and within the brain substance. Variable enhancement is encountered following contrast infusion.

Orbital implants are well outlined by CT. Extrusion or displacement of an implant indicates recurrent tumor in the orbit. Regression of tumor following radiation and chemotherapy can also be assessed by CT.

CAVERNOUS HEMANGIOMA OF THE RETINA AND OPTIC NERVE

This vascular hamartoma is familial and is encountered in association with one or more intracranial cavernous hemangiomas, as well as angiomatous hamartomas of the skin and other organs.[18,19] The hemangioma is composed of thin-walled, sacular aneurysms filled with dark, venous blood. The disease appears to be inherited as an autosomal dominant. The lesion has the appearance of grapes projecting from the inner surface of the optic nerve and retina.

CEREBRAL ANGIOMATOSIS: VON HIPPEL-LINDAU'S DISEASE

This disease is characterized by benign capillary tumors manifested by elevated red masses, which may arise anywhere in the retina or optic nerve.[20–22] They are bilateral in 50 percent of cases. They are inherited as an autosomal dominant trait and may be associated in approximately 25 percent of cases with similar vascular hamartomas in the central nervous system, predominantly cerebellum, midbrain, and spinal cord. The tumor may arise from the inner (endophytic) or outer (exophytic) retinal layers. If the tumor reaches a certain size, the artery and vein supplying and draining the tumor dilate and become tortuous. In all the lesions, the capillaries comprising the tumor become incompetent and cause intraretinal and subretinal transudation, hemorrhage, and exudation. The visual function of these patients is normal until they develop intra- and subretinal exudation.

CONGENITAL RETINAL ARTERIOVENOUS MALFORMATION: WYBURN-MASON SYNDROME

This malformation affects primarily the major retinal vessels. It is usually unilateral and may be confined to one portion of the retina and optic nerve head or may involve the entire retina.[23] The retinal vessels are dilated, tortuous, and often more numerous than normal. Hemorrhage and exudation into the retina are frequent. The lesion may be familial. The degree of visual loss is variable and parallels the extent of the vascular anomaly. The retinal malformations may be associated with similar ipsilateral malformations of the face, orbit, optic nerve, maxilla, pterygoid fossa, mandible and frontal area, sylvian fissure, posterior fossa, and midbrain. Wyburn-Mason emphasized the association of retinal and midbrain vascular malformations.

TUBEROUS SCLEROSIS *(Case 15)*

Ocular involvement in tuberous sclerosis is characterized by white retinal glial hamartomatous tumors, which may be single, multiple, flat and smooth or raised with a cobblestone appearance.[24] Both retinal and intracranial lesions may calcify in time.

Other than the described ocular findings, this disease is characterized by adenoma sebaceum, mental retardation, and epilepsy. The disease is inherited as an irregular dominant trait with high penetrance and variable expressivity.

ENCEPHALOTRIGEMINAL ANGIOMATOSIS: STURGE-WEBER'S DISEASE

This syndrome is characterized by intracranial, facial, and choroidal angiomas, all homolateral and present from birth.[25] There is no evidence that the disease is inherited. The intracranial hemangioma involves the meninges and exhibits fine parallel lines of calcification. There is often associated unilateral atrophy of the cerebral cortex. There may be seizures, visual field defects, and mental deficiency.

On the same side as the central nervous system lesions, there are cutaneous angiomas (nervous flammeus) that follow the distribution of the first and second division of the fifth nerve. The lesion almost always involves the lid and palpebral and bulbar conjunctiva. Facial hemihypertrophy of the involved side is not infrequent. In the eye, the choroidal hemangioma is reflected by a darker choroid. CT demonstrates the choroidal hemangioma, manifesting as an enhancing, thickened choroidal rim. Retro-ocular hemangiomas may also be present (see Chapter 6, Case 5). Other eye findings are glaucoma, dilation and tortuosity of conjunctival vessels, and heterochromia iridis.

NEUROFIBROMATOSIS

This is a congenital disorder inherited through a regular or irregular dominant gene that varies markedly in its expression. The following findings are encountered[26–28]:

1. flat, light brown café-au-lait spots varying in size with irregular borders and best seen on the trunk
2. subcutaneous tumors
3. skeletal changes
4. orbital dysplasia
5. occasional mental retardation
6. associated intracranial tumors such as glioma, meningioma, and acoustic neurinoma

The eye lesions consist of plexiform or pedunculated neurofibromas of the lids, conjunctiva, cornea, iris, choroid, and retina. Congenital glaucoma may also be associated with neurofibromatosis. The bony orbital dysplasia, tumors of the anterior visual pathway, orbital neurofibromas, and large ocular bulbs are all well demonstrated by CT (see Chapter 3, Cases 6–17).

CHOROIDAL OSTEOMA *(Cases 15–21)*

Choroidal osteomas are composed of cancellous bone and arise in the juxtapapillary choroid in female patients.[29,30] The patients are usually asymptomatic until late childhood, when they present with central or paracentral scotoma. The lesions cause elevation of the retina and appear orange to orange-white with sharply defined margins. These tumors may simulate a choroidal hemangioma. However, the sharp border distinguishes it from a hemangioma. If the tumor reaches a certain size, retinal detachment and choroidal neovascularization are seen. Histologically, the tumor is composed of mature bone with a hypocellular marrow. The lesion occurs predominantly in females, but can also occur in males. Choroidal osteoma has to be differentiated from lesions that are calcified. The differential diagnosis of calcifications of the posterior globe includes the following:

Differential Diagnosis of Calcific Densities of the Posterior Globe[31,32]

1. Primary neural tumors of the retina and optic nerve
   Retinoblastoma
   Optic nerve glioma
   Optic nerve meningioma
2. Glial hamartomas of the optic nerve and retina
   Tuberous sclerosis
   von Recklinghausen's disease
   Drusen
   Isolated
3. Vascular tumors of the retina and choroid
   Cavernous hemangioma
   Hemangioendothelioma
   Choroidal osteoma
4. Hypercalcemic states
   Hyperparathyroidism
   Hypervitaminosis D
   Sarcoidosis
   Hypercalcemia of chronic renal disease

5. Posttraumatic, postinflammatory, degenerative conditions

   Phthisis bulbi

   Retrolental fibroplasia

CT of a choroidal osteoma reveals a lesion with bone density most often located in the posterior pole. The lesion is usually round or oval in shape and sharply marginated. It may be single or multiple in one globe, or arise bilaterally. The remaining structures in the eye are usually normal. The calcification seen on CT scanning distinguishes choroidal osteoma from amelanotic melanoma, metastatic carcinoma, leukemic or lymphomatous infiltrates—which may be difficult to differentiate on fundoscopic examination.

STAPHYLOMA *(Cases 22 and 23)*

A staphyloma represents a localized or generalized scleral ectasia with uveal tissue present within the ectatic cavity.[34] According to anatomic location, one differentiates the lesion as follows:

1. anterior staphyloma—between ciliary body and cornea
2. ciliary staphyloma—over ciliary body
3. equatorial staphyloma—at globe equator
4. posterior staphyloma—between equator and optic nerve

Partial staphylomas are caused by increased intraocular pressure, local decrease in the resistance of the sclera to stress caused by injuries or inflammation of the sclera. Posterior staphyloma are often the result of severe and prolonged glaucoma with optic atrophy or a high degree of myopia. CT is able to demonstrate the location and size of the ectasia.

BUPHTHALMOS *(Case 24)*

Buphthalmia, or primary infantile glaucoma, is caused by increased intraocular pressure, which has its onset in the first three years of life, with 80 percent manifest by age one.[33] It is inherited through an autosomal recessive gene.

The findings, in order of their occurrence in increasing severity are:

1. photophobia
2. lacrimation
3. blepharospasm
4. corneal haziness and enlargement
5. rupture of Descemet's membrane and glaucomatous cupping of the optic nerve

If the condition is untreated, the eye enlarges and may rupture. CT demonstrates a diffusely enlarged globe. The condition may be bilateral.

MICROPHTHALMOS *(Case 25)*

Microphthalmos is inherited as either a dominant or recessive autosomal trait. In pure microphthalmia, the eye is normal, but two-thirds of its proper size. It can be unilateral, but is usually bilateral. Frequently, there are other associated ocular defects. Microphthalmia may be part of various systemic abnormalities.[33] It is frequently associated with a congenital serous cyst, which may in fact, enlarge the orbit. It appears that these so-called colobomatous orbitopalpebral cysts may communicate with the eye and are associated with a defective closure of the embryonic cleft.

PHTHISIS BULBI *(Case 26)*

Phthisis bulbi refers to a shrinkage of the eye, which is usually a sequela of severe longstanding ophthalmic disease with degeneration. The pathologic process follows different conditions, including trauma with an intraocular foreign body, rupture of the globe, or longstanding ocular inflammatory disease. The structures of the eye are disorganized, atrophic, and shrunken. The terminal process is characterized by ossification and/or calcification of the choroid, ciliary body, and cyclitic membrane. These calcifications are often crescent-shaped and follow the outline of the choroid.[31,35] Calcification of the lens may develop as a consequence of the degenerative process. CT is able to demonstrate the shrunken, deformed globe and the calcific densities.

MISCELLANEOUS CASES *(Cases 27–29)*

Other disorders are illustrated in Cases 27–29.

REFERENCES

1. Cancer Facts and Figures 1980. New York, American Cancer Society, 1979
2. Brady LW, Shields JA, Augsburger TJ, Day JL: Malignant intraocular tumors. Cancer 49:578–585, 1982
3. del Regato JA, Spjut HJ: Cancer of the eye. In Cancer—Diagnosis, Treatment, Prognosis, 5th ed. St. Louis, CV Mosby, 1977, pp 160–181
4. Stephens RF, Shields JA: Diagnosis and management of cancer metastatic to the uvea: a study of 70 cases. Ophthalmology 86:1336–1349, 1979
5. Shields JA, Zimmerman LE: Lesions simulating malignant melanoma of the posterior uvea. Arch Ophthalmol 89:466–471, 1973
6. Gass JDM: Differential Diagnosis of Intraocular Tumors. St. Louis, CV Mosby, 1974, pp. 59–105
7. Rones B, Zimmerman LE: An unusual choroidal hemorrhage simulating malignant melanoma. Arch Ophthalmol 70:30–32, 1963
8. Bernardino ME, Danziger J, Young SE, Wallace S: Computed tomography in ocular neoplastic disease. AJR 131:111–113, 1978

9. Starr HJ, Zimmerman LE: Extrascleral extension and orbital recurrence of malignant melanomas of the choroid and ciliary body. Int Ophthalmol Clin 2:369–385, 1962

10. Kitchen FD: Genetics of retinoblastoma. In Reese AB (ed): Tumors of the Eye. New York, Harper & Row, 1976, pp. 125–132

11. Mokely TA Jr: Retinoblastoma in a 52-year-old man. Arch Ophthalmol 69:325–327, 1963

12. Reese AB: Retinoblastoma and other neuroectodermal tumors of the retina. In Reese AB (ed): Tumors of the Eye. New York, Harper & Row, 1976, pp. 90–124

13. Rootman J, Hofbauer J, Ellsworth RM, Kitchen D: A clinicopathological study of optic nerve invasion by retinoblastoma. Read before the Canadian Ophthalmological Society, June 1975

14. Jones IS, Jakobiek FA (eds): Diseases of the Orbit. Hagerstown, Md., Harper & Row, 1979, p 504

15. Danziger A, Price H: CT findings in retinoblastoma. AJR 133:695–697, 1979

16. Goldberg L, Danziger A: Computed tomographic scanning in the management of retinoblastoma. Am J Ophthalmol 84:380–382, 1977

17. Zimmerman R, Belaniuk L: Computed tomography in the evaluation of patients with bilateral retinoblastomas. CT: J Comput Tomogr 3:251–257, 1979

18. Davies WS, Thumin M: Cavernous hemangioma of the optic disc and retina. Trans Am Acad Ophalmal Otolargyngol 60:217–218, 1956

19. Lewis RA, Cohen MH, Wise GN: Cavernous hemangioma of the retina and optic disc. A report of three cases and a review of the literature. Br J Ophthal 59:422–434, 1975

20. Melmon KL, Rosen SW: Lindau's disease. Review of the literature and study of a large kindred. Am J Med 36:595–617, 1964

21. Goldberg MF, Koenig S: Argon laser treatment of von Hippel-Lindau retinal angiomas. I. Clinical and angiographic findings. Arch Opththalmol 92:121–125, 1974

22. Welch RB: Von Hippel-Lindau disease: The recognition and treatment of early angiomatosis retinae and the use of cryosurgery as an adjunct to therapy. Trans Am Ophthalmol Soc 68:367–424, 1970

23. Wyburn-Mason R: Arteriovenous aneurysm of midbrain and retina, facial naevi and mental changes, Brain 66:163–203, 1943

24. McLean JM: Glial tumors of the retina in relation to tuberous sclerosis. Am J Ophthalmol 41:428–432, 1956

25. Alexander GL, Norman RM: The Sturge-Weber Syndrome. Bristol, UK, John Wright, 1960, 95

26. Jacoby CG, Go RT, Beren RA: Cranial CT of neurofibromatosis. AJNR 1:311–315, 1980

27. Casselman ES, Miller WT, Lin SR, Mandell GA: Von Recklinghaussen's disease: incidence of roentgenographic findings with a clinical review of the literature. CRC Crit Rev Diagn Imag 9:387–419, 1977

28. Klatte EC, Franken EA, Smith JA: The radiographic spectrum in neurofibromatosis. Semin Roentgenol 11:17–33, 1976

29. Laibovitz R: An unusual case of intraocular calcification: choroidal osteoma. Ann Ophthalmol 11:1077–1080, 1979

30. Gass JDM: Choroidal osteoma. Arch Ophthalmol 96:428–435, 1978

31. Brant-Zawadzki M, Enzmann D: Orbital computed tomography: calcific densities of the posterior globe. J Comput Assist Tomogr 3:503–505, 1979

32. Edwards MK, Buncic JR, Harwood-Nash DC: Optic disc drusen. J Comput Assist Tomogr 6:383–384, 1982

33. Duke-Elder WS (ed): Systems of Ophthalmology, Vol 3. St. Louis, CV Mosby, 1963, pp 488–495

34. Scheie HG, Albert D: Textbook of Ophthalmology, 9th ed. Philadelphia, Saunders, 1977, pp 21–22

35. Duke-Elder WS (ed): Systems of Ophthalmology, Vol 7, St. Louis, CV Mosby, 1962, pp 180–182

CASE 1. Malignant Melanoma
A 71-year-old male with a 1-week history of blurred vision and redness of right eye. A black spot was noted when elevating the right lid.

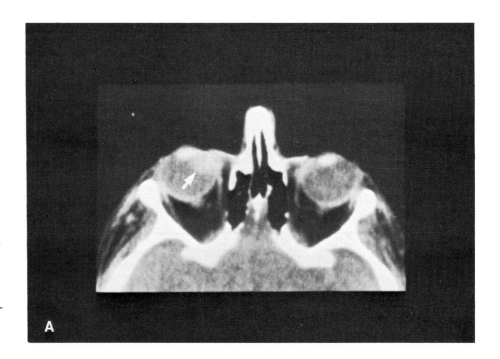

Figure A. A soft-tissue mass occupies the nasal quadrant of the globe (arrow). The mass is contiguous with the lens, ciliary body, and global rim. There is slight deformity of the rim anteromedially, suggesting scleral invasion.

Follow-up: The patient underwent right orbital exenteration. Pathologic examination revealed an invasive malignant uveal melanoma, spindle cell B type, involving the ciliary body, peripheral choroid and iris, with extrascleral extension into the subconjunctival space. The optic nerve and adenexa were uninvolved.

CASE 2. Malignant Melanoma

A 62-year-old female with visual loss on left. Fundoscopy revealed a pigmented choroidal mass. A P32 uptake test was positive.

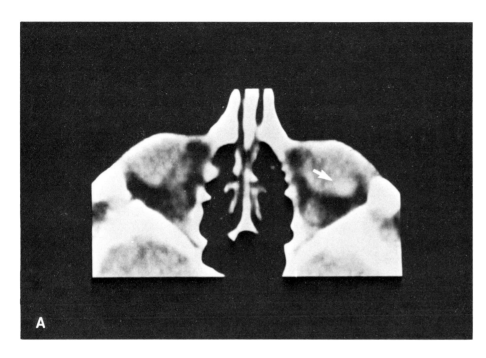

Figure A. CT demonstrates an eccentrically placed mass extending into the vitreous chamber (arrow). There is deformity of the adjacent scleral rim, suggesting invasion.

Follow-up: The exenterated specimen revealed extraocular tumor extension.

CASE 3. Malignant Melanoma

A cataract was removed from the right eye of this 91-year-old female a year earlier. She has had progressive right proptosis for three months. Examination revealed 13 mm of proptosis OD with marked increased orbital resistance and no extraocular movement. A mass was palpable in the lower fornix. Vision, 20/60 OS, no light perception OD.

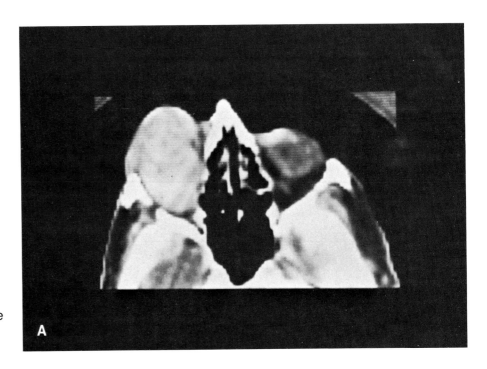

Figure A. Marked right proptosis is present. The globe is uniformly dense, indicating that it is completely filled with tumor. The entire retro-ocular space is occupied by mass.

Follow-up: At surgery, a choroidal melanoma that had extensively invaded the globe and retrobulbar area was found. An orbital exenteration was performed, but residual tumor in the orbital apex remained.

CASE 4. Malignant Melanoma

An 83-year-old male with a pigmented nodule in the left orbit. He had a history of cataract extractions and open-angle glaucoma.

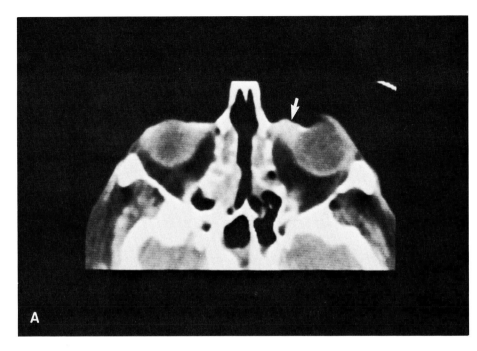

Figure A. A contrast scan demonstrates a contrast-enhancing mass (arrow) in the anterior medial aspect of the left orbit. The mass does not appear to extend posteriorly beyond the orbital septum. The globe is displaced laterally. Incidental note is made of membrane thickening and opacification of the ethmoid sinuses.

Follow-up: A biopsy revealed malignant melanoma. This was followed by radiation therapy.

CASE 5. Orbital Exenteration
This 60-year-old male had metastatic melanoma to the right globe and optic nerve that required a right orbital exenteration.

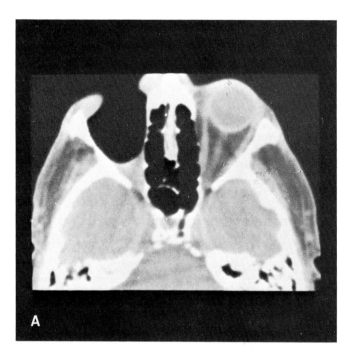 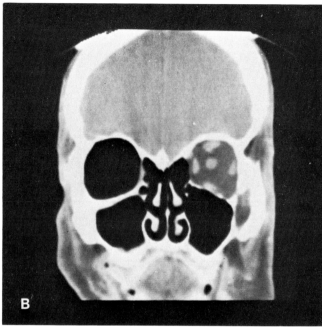

Figures A and B. Axial and coronal scans show the right orbital exenteration. The globe, optic nerve, and all the extraocular muscles have been removed. A small amount of soft tissue remains in the apex of the orbit.

Follow-up: Despite the orbital exenteration, the patient later developed additional metastases to the ribs and iliac crest.

CASE 6. Bilateral Retinoblastoma

This three-month-old male presented with bilateral leukocoria.

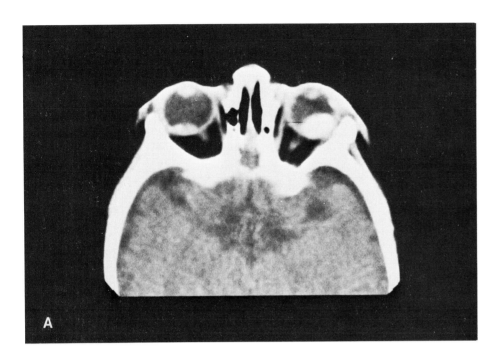

Figure A. Bilateral ocular calcifications are noted, more extensive on the left. There is no evidence of retro-ocular invasion, and the optic nerves appear normal.

Follow-up: Metastatic workup was negative. Therapy involved 4800 rad delivered to each eye. Examination subsequently revealed residual dead tumors occupying both macular areas.

CASE 7. Bilateral Retinoblastoma

A newborn infant female with positive family history for bilateral retinoblastoma, found at birth to have bilateral leukocoria and retinoblastoma.

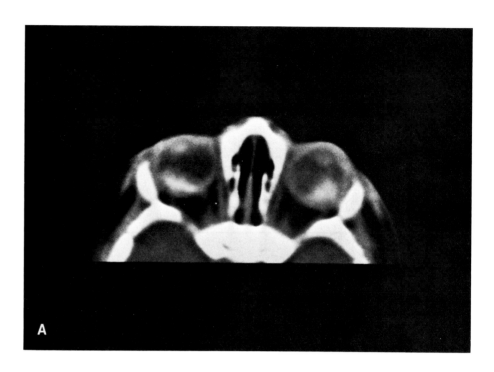

Figure A. Bilateral ocular calcification occupying the posterior poles of the globes are present. On the left the tumor appears more extensive, almost involving the lens. No retro-ocular invasion is noted.

A

Follow-up: The patient was treated with radiation, 4600 rad delivered to each eye over 39 days. Subsequent examination revealed that the tumors had shrunk down to a fourth of their original size. However, she developed progressive rubeosis iridis, which necessitated bilateral enucleation. Pathologic examination revealed necrotic retinoblastomas secondary to the radiation therapy, with no choroidal or optic nerve involvement. Preretinal fibrovascular membranes, retinal cystic changes, and traction retinal detachments were present.

CASE 8. Bilateral Retinoblastoma

A three-month-old female with two-week history of the left eye wandering. The mother noted a white reflex from the left pupil. Examination revealed left-sided leukocoria with a white subretinal mass and total retinal detachment. The right eye revealed a white gelatinous exophytic mass above the macula. The family history was negative for retinoblastoma.

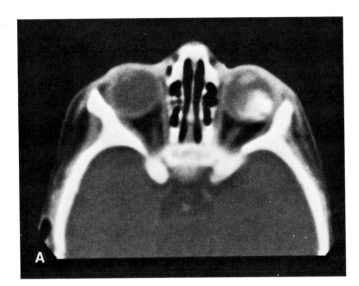 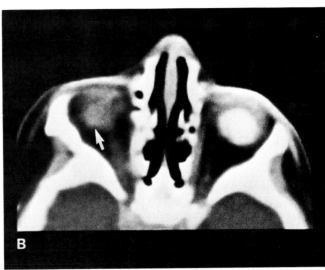

Figures A and B. CT demonstrates a large left ocular mass that is partially calcified. The retrobulbar structures are normal. No definite abnormality of the right eye could be demonstrated. The ill-defined density on the right (arrow) could be the tumor.

Follow-up: The left eye was enucleated. The right eye was treated with 4500 rad over five weeks.

CASE 9. Retinoblastoma

A nine-month-old male with three-month history of left eye deviation and abnormal pupil. Leukocoria and acute glaucoma were present at examination.

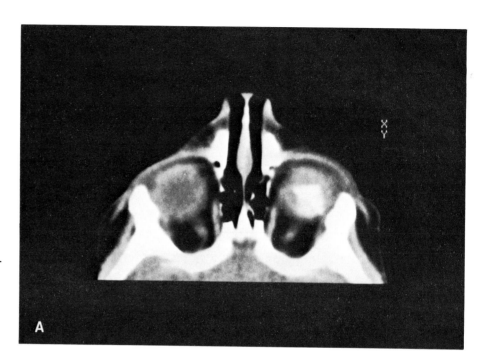

Figure A. A calcified mass is present involving the left globe. The tumor extends beyond the calcification and manifests as a diffuse increase in density occupying the entire globe.

Follow-up: The eye was enucleated.

CASE 10. Bilateral Retinoblastoma

This one-year-old infant's mother noted deviation of the left eye for one month. Abnormal pupillary color was recently noted.

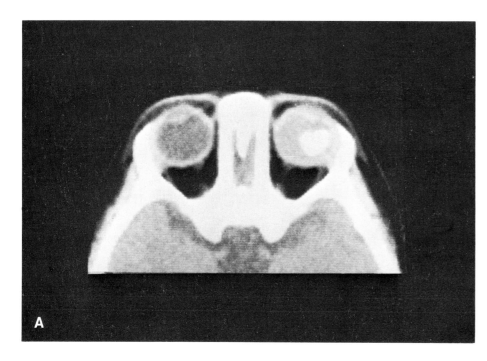

Figure A. The left ocular calcification occupies much of the vitreous chamber. The remainder of the globe is filled with soft-tissue density representing noncalcified tumor. In a more craniad CT section, a small calcified density, representing the right retinoblastoma, was identified (not illustrated).

Follow-up: The left eye was enucleated. The right side was treated with radiation.

CASE 11. Retinoblastoma

A 17-month-old female with deviation of left eye. Also, recent history of frequent falling and bumping into things. A subretinal mass with a detached retina was present on the left. Ultrasound examination revealed a mass with high internal echos. The right eye was normal.

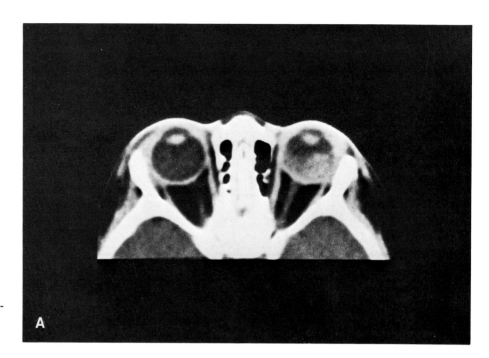

Figure A. A left-sided mass is present, entirely within the confines of the globe. No obvious calcification is present within the mass.

Follow-up: The left eye was enucleated. There was no invasion of the choroid or sclera.

CASE 12. Recurrent Retinoblastoma

This 3-year-old male presented with strabismus of left eye at age 1½ years. He underwent left eye enucleation. Pathologic examination revealed a high-grade retinoblastoma involving the optic nerve with negative resection margins. There was extensive choroidal involvement. No postoperative radiation therapy was given. He recently was noted to have multiple small conjunctival nodules, which revealed recurrent retinoblastoma on biopsy. There was no evidence of systemic spread.

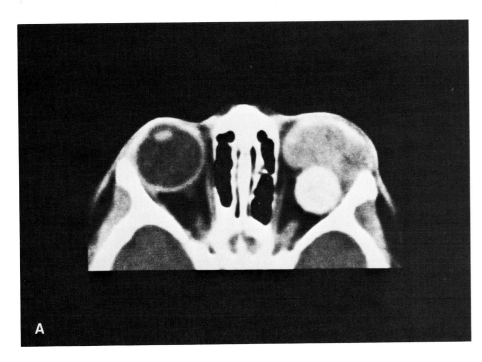

A

Figure A. A soft-tissue mass representing the recurrent tumor occupies the anterior left globe, displacing the dense prosthesis posteriorly. There is no bony destruction. There was no evidence of intracranial spread on further CT examination.

Follow-up: The patient was referred for emergency radiation of the left orbit and subsequent chemotherapy.

CASE 13. Bilateral Retinoblastoma

A nine-month-old female with positive family history of retinoblastoma presented with a white right pupil. Examination revealed bilateral retinoblastomas. She subsequently underwent right-sided enucleation and 4000 rad radiation therapy over three weeks to the left eye. Subsequent retinal detachments on the left were treated with cryocoagulation and xenon arc photocoagulation. Further detachments were treated with a scleral buckle procedure. Drainage of the subretinal fluid revealed no malignant cells. Her course has been further complicated by the development of a subcapsular cataract.

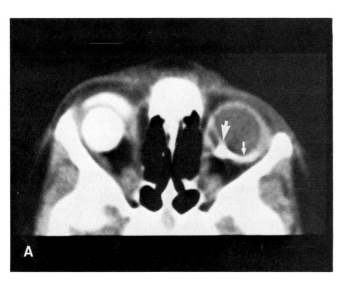 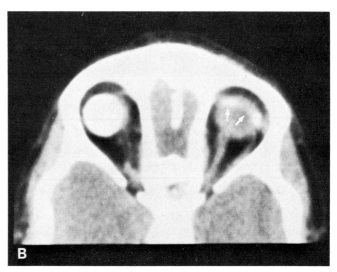

Figure A. A right-sided prosthesis is present. On the left, the rounded dense calcification (large arrow) represents the residual treated retinoblastoma. Adjacent to it, the curvilinear calcification is the encircling band from the scleral buckle procedure (small arrow).

Figure B. CT section craniad to A again demonstrates the circumferential band (arrows).

CASE 14. Bilateral Retinal Dysplasia

A one-month-old male found on well-baby examination to have bilateral leu-kocoria. No family history of retinoblastoma. Examination under anesthesia with indirect ophthalmoscopy revealed a solid-appearing mass lesion on the left with no retinal structures visualized. On the right, several whitish masses were identified within the vitreous cavity. Evaluation by ultrasonography did not reveal strong evidence of a solid-mass lesion in either eye. The diagnostic possibilities of a uveitis versus retinoblastoma were considered.

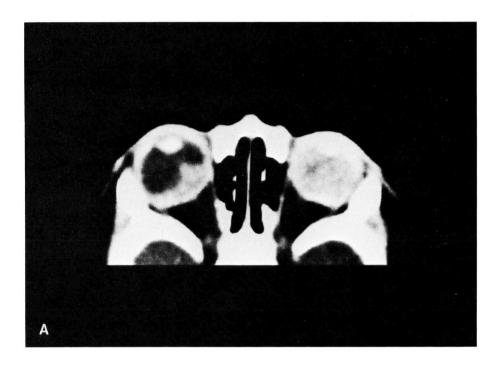

Figure A. The left globe is filled with a soft-tissue mass, without calcification. The apparent increased density of the lesion is due to the narrow window. On the right, a soft-tissue mass protrudes into the vitreous chamber. The retro-ocular areas are bilaterally normal.

Follow-up: The left eye was enucleated. Pathologic examination revealed retinal dysplasia and retinal detachment without evidence of retinoblastoma.

CASE 15. Tuberous Sclerosis
This 15-year-old male with tuberous sclerosis presented with visual loss on the right. Fundoscopy revealed a small white retinal nodule.

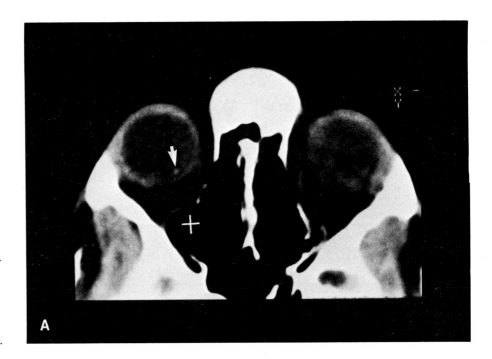

Figure A. There is a small calcification in the posterior right globe (arrow) consistent with a hamartomatous lesion. The calcification, however, is nonspecific. No intracranial calcifications were present.

CASES 16 to 18. Choroidal Osteomas

Three young females presented with visual loss. Fundoscopy demonstrated the characteristic yellow-white color of choroidal osteomas.

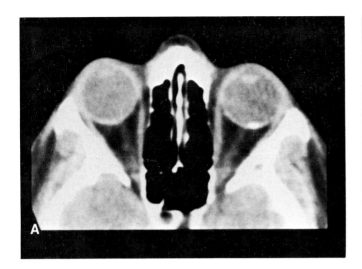

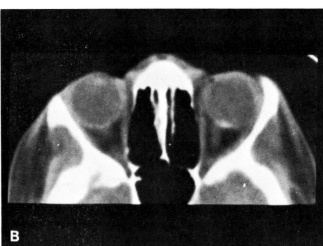

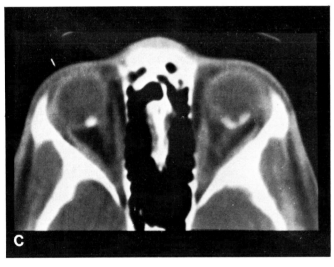

Figures A–C. Unilateral and bilateral posterior globe discrete calcifications are present. The calcifications are nonspecific, but together with the clinical findings, they are consistent with choroidal osteomas.

CASE 19. Hyperparathyroidism with Ocular Calcification
A 38-year-old male with hypercalcemia due to hyperparathyroidism.

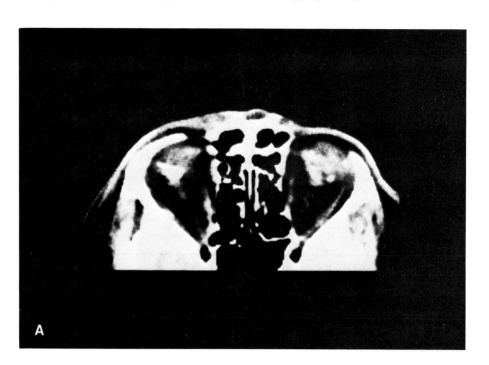

Figure A. CT section through the upper orbit demonstrates extensive bilateral ocular calcifications.

CASE 20. Sarcoidosis with Ocular Calcifications

A 74-year-old female status postsurgery for detached retina on the right 10 years previously. Long history of sarcoidosis with hypercalcemia. She had been treated with vitamin D in the past. Presented with gout and a macula mass on the right. Vision: 20/20 OS, 20/40 OD.

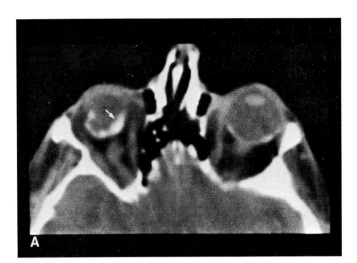 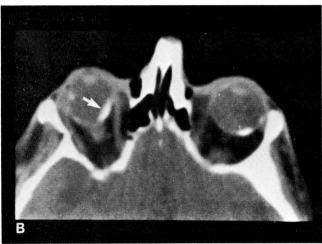

Figures A and B. Bilateral ocular calcifications are present, presumably secondary to the sarcoidosis. The oval shape of the right globe is due to the previous scleral buckle procedure. The curvilinear density on the right (arrow) represents part of the scleral band.

CASE 21. Nocardia of Choroid

This 26-year-old female with T-cell lymphoma, controlled on chemotherapy, developed rapid onset of left-sided visual loss. Fundoscopy revealed an elevated lesion adjacent to macula. Nocardia was isolated from a lung biopsy.

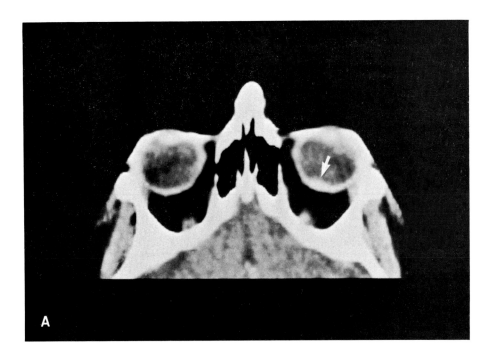

Figure A. The choroidal lesion is seen as a focal thickening of the ocular rim projecting slightly into the vitreous (arrow).

CASE 22. Staphyloma: Calcified Lens

A 78-year-old female who 14 years before had developed right facial herpes zoster. Within two weeks she was completely blind with opacification of the cornea. She presented with enlargement and darkening of the right eye. In view of the possibility of an intraocular melanoma, enucleation was performed.

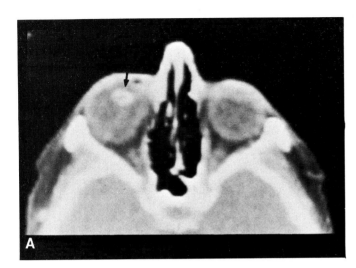 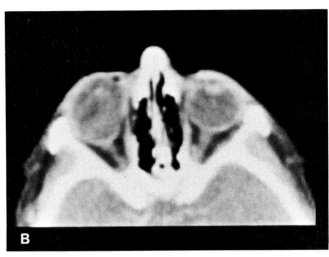

Figures A and B. The right globe is enlarged with asymmetrical bulges involving the perimeter. There is calcification of the lens (arrow) involving the capsule primarily. The central part of the lens remains lucent.

Follow-up: Pathologic examination of the enucleated globe revealed two large staphylomatous bulges. No melanoma was present.

CASE 23. Staphyloma

This 30-year-old female with Down's syndrome presented with headache. Retinoscopy documented a severe right myopia. Fundoscopy revealed asymmetric bulging of the posterior globe with increased pigmentation of the involved choroid.

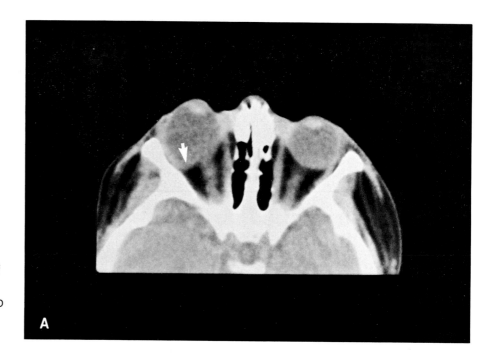

Figure A. The right globe is enlarged with asymmetric bulging of the posterior pole. At the site of the focal ectasia, there appears to be a deficiency of the scleral rim (arrow).

CASE 24. Congenital Buphthalmos
This two-year-old infant presented with bilateral prominent eyes.

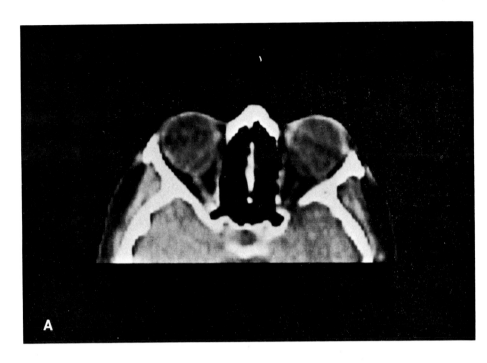

A

Figure A. The pseudoproptosis results from symmetrically enlarged ocular bulbs secondary to the congenital glaucoma.

CASE 25. Microphthalmos with Congenital Retrobulbar Cyst

A seven-month-old female who was noted at birth to have severe bilateral ocular anomalies. The blind right eye was proptotic but small in size and with a reduced anterior segment and retinal detachments. The left eye revealed iris and choroidal colobomata with involvement of the disc and macula.

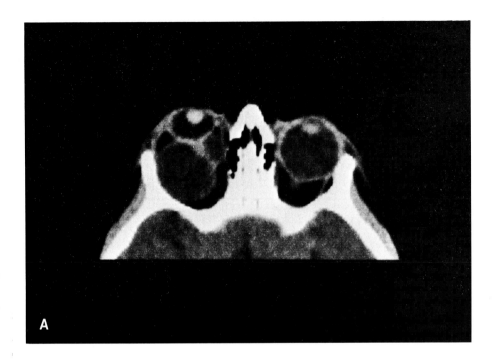

Figure A. The right orbit is enlarged with an increased transverse diameter and outward bowing of the lateral wall. The ocular bulb is small and is displaced forward by a large retrobulbar cyst. The cyst appears loculated.

CASE 26. Phthisis Bulbi

A 67-year-old male with a 12-year history of left-sided uveitis (idiopathic). Subsequently developed bulbous keratopathy. Management included corneal transplant, cataract extraction, peripheral iridectomy, and cryotherapy. He had progressive loss of vision. Patient declined enucleation.

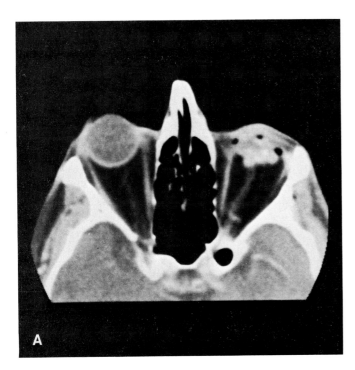 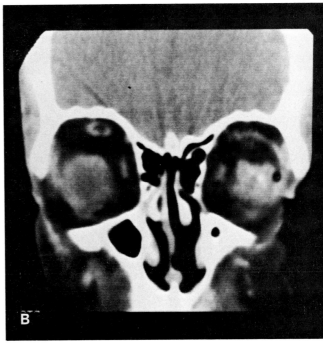

Figures A and B. Axial and coronal sections demonstrate the characteristic changes of phthisis bulbi, with a shrunken, irregular, atrophic globe containing calcium flecks.

CASE 27. Status Post-insertion of Scleral Buckle and Encircling Band
A 52-year-old female who, several years previously, had a successful scleral buckle procedure for a left-sided retinal detachment. In addition, she had several transcranial surgical procedures to repair a recurrent CSF rhinorrhea. These images of the orbit were obtained during a CT metrizamide cisternogram to localize the site of the CSF leak.

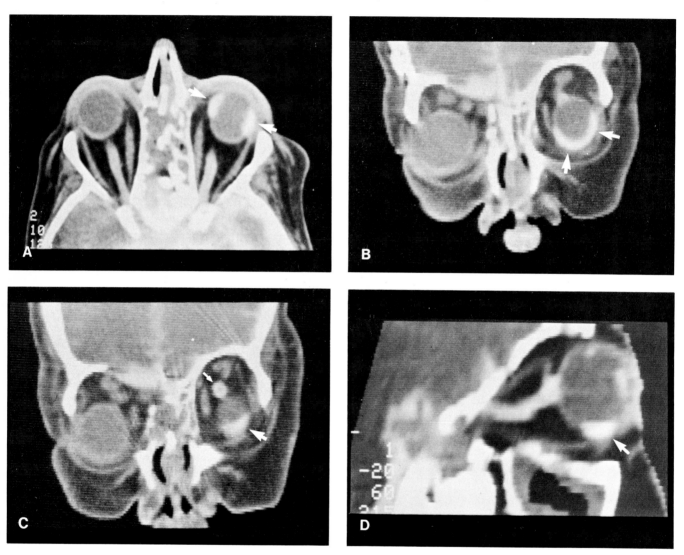

Figures A–D. Axial, coronal, and sagittal views of the orbit demonstrate the residuum of a scleral buckle procedure. The left globe has an oval configuration, with demonstration of the circumferential band (large arrows). Note that the metrizamide had filled the perioptic subarachnoid spaces bilaterally. The optic nerve is seen as a central lucency, particularly in C (small arrow).

CASE 28. Hypertelorism: Rudimentary Extraocular Muscles

Female child with congenital bilateral external ophthalmoplegia and bilateral ptosis. Hypertelorism was present. Vision: 20/20 OU.

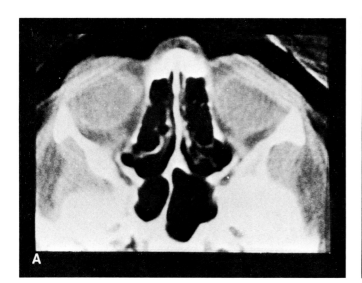 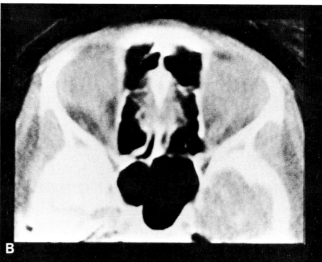

Figures A and B. The ocular bulbs are bilaterally enlarged, occupying most of the orbital spaces. Very small, rudimentary extraocular muscles can be identified. The optic nerves appear normal. The internasal distance is increased.

Follow-up: Surgery was performed on the left for strabismus. No extraocular muscles were found.

CASE 29. Basal Cell Carcinoma of Sebaceous Gland
This is a 70-year-old female with an ulcerating, slowly enlarging right orbital mass for 2 years.

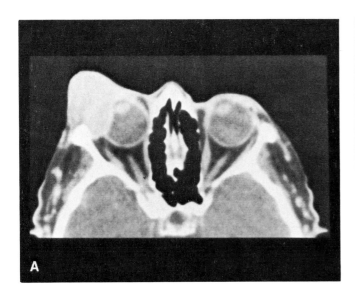
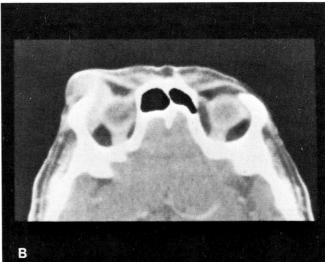

Figures A and B. CT scans show a large contrast-enhancing mass in the anterior lateral aspect of the right orbit. The mass deforms the anterior lateral aspect of the globe and displaces the globe medially. The retrobulbar region is free of tumor, and no bone erosion is evident.

Follow-up: A biopsy of the mass revealed sebaceous cell carcinoma. A right orbital exenteration was performed with dissection of the lateral bony wall.

CHAPTER NINE

Trauma

Computed tomography is helpful in the evaluation of complex orbital and facial trauma because it provides visualization of soft tissues, bony structures, and foreign bodies.[1-3] Advances in CT technology have allowed very thin section scanning, thereby improving spatial resolution. Newer software packages allow greater flexibility of data manipulation, permitting image reformation in multiple planes. Axial and coronal 5-mm contiguous sections are the baseline study for evaluation of maxillofacial trauma. Multiplanar image reformation in combination with thin 1.5-mm axial sections is an alternative method for studying traumatized patients. This has the advantage of not subjecting the patient to the hyperextended head position required for direct coronals, as well as allowing sagittal images of the orbital floor to be obtained. These are necessary to evaluate blowout fractures. In newer scanners, the rapid time (2 seconds) allows the examination of the acutely injured but stable patient to be performed in a relatively short period of time. Intracranial and cervical spine injuries can be assessed simultaneously with the facial and orbital trauma.[4-6] Up to 30 percent of cases of significant facial and orbital trauma are associated with head injuries.

Plain film examinations and complex tomography have been the standard for radiologic diagnosis of maxillo–orbital fractures. However, in complex orbitofacial trauma, CT provides the most effective imaging modality. The superior contrast resolution of CT allows easier identification of displaced fragments, thus representing the ideal imaging modality for complex fractures such as LeFort II and III.

Contrast enhancement is not routinely utilized but may be necessary in suspected vascular injuries such as caroticocavernous fistula.[7]

CT metrizamide cisternography has become the procedure of choice in the determination of the site of a CSF leak. These leaks may originate from the sphenoid sinus, cribriform-ethmoidal area, and posterior wall of the frontal sinus. Both axial and coronal views are often required in the evaluation of these cases. The coronal views are required to study the roof of the ethmoid labyrinth, the cribriform plates, and the roof of the sphenoid sinus. At the time of the study, there should be active CSF leakage.

The following parameters should be assessed by CT in patients with orbitofacial trauma:

1. number and exact location of fractures
2. degree and direction of fracture displacement
3. demonstration of detached bony fragments within the orbital cavity and adjacent intracranial cavity
4. evaluation of soft-tissue injury
5. assessment of damage to the intraorbital contents, including globe, muscle prolapse or entrapment, optic nerve transection and hematoma formation, and orbital emphysema
6. traumatic meningoencephalocele in the sinuses, orbit, or nasal cavity

In cases of suspected intracranial injuries, a search should be made for extradural-subdural hematoma, brain contusion, or pneumocephalus.

CT is not without limitations, however. Coronal CT is uncomfortable and often impossible to perform in a severely injured patient. It is contraindicated when a cervical spine injury is suspected. Artifacts caused by dental fillings and bullets appear as radial streaks on coronal views and may obscure fracture fragments and foreign bodies. Polytomography, by virtue of its slightly better spatial resolution has been superior to CT scanning, especially for fine bone detail. However, in general, this is more than compensated for by the greater contrast resolution of CT.

TYPES OF FRACTURES

Isolated Fractures

Isolated fractures may involve the inferior and superior orbital rim, lateral wall of the orbit, maxillary and zygomatic bone, maxillary sinus, or zygomatic arch. These fractures are best evaluated by conventional facial films and, in some instances, polytomography.

Orbital roof fractures, with or without frontal sinus fractures, however, are better identified on CT, which may require imaging in the axial and coronal planes. Brain contusion may accompany orbital roof fractures.

Zygomaticomaxillary Fractures *(Cases 1 and 2)*
This type of fracture reveals the following findings:

1. Increased soft-tissue density over the face and orbit, together with variable opacification of the maxillary sinus, nasal cavity, and ethmoid sinus on the involved side. This usually stems from blood or edema and is occasionally associated with a fluid level in the maxillary sinus.
2. Separation of frontozygomatic suture or a horizontal fracture above or below the suture.
3. Fracture of the inferior orbital rim.
4. Fracture of the lateral-posterior wall of the maxillary sinus and occasionally an anterior wall fracture.
5. Fracture of the orbital floor—this fracture may be slight and clinically insignificant. However, a severe blow to the face may produce a floor fracture with marked comminution, superior buckling, or marked depression.
6. Fracture in the zygomatic arch with slight to severe depression and occasionally outward buckling.

There may be an associated vertical or oblique fracture in the zygomatic or maxillary bones, usually at the suture of these two bones.

In most zygomaticomaxillary fractures, assessment by conventional films and polytomography will suffice. In severe floor fractures with ptosis of the globe, muscle entrapment, and/or optic nerve injury, CT may be useful. The degree of rotation and displacement is easily evaluated.

LeFort II Fracture (Pyramidal Fracture)
The following findings are encountered:

1. increased density in the maxillary and sometimes ethmoid and frontal sinuses
2. fracture of the nasal bones, frontal process of maxillae, lamina papyracea, and lacrimal bones bilaterally
3. fracture of the inferior rim and floor of both orbits
4. fracture near or through zygomaticomaxillary suture
5. deformity or discontinuity of the lateral wall of the maxillary sinuses
6. fracture through the pterygoid processes
7. involvement of frontal and ethmoid sinuses in approximately 10 percent of cases

LeFort III Fracture (Craniofacial Disjunction) *(Cases 3 and 4)*
The following findings are demonstrated:

1. severe facial swelling with increased density in all sinuses
2. diastasis of the zygomaticofrontal, maxillofrontal, and nasofrontal sutures
3. posterior extension of fractures to include the cribriform plates, ethmoid labyrinth, and possibly the body of sphenoid
4. fracture through the pterygoid processes

LeFort II and III fractures are best evaluated by CT in the axial and coronal planes. In these complex-type fractures, significant soft-tissue injuries, opacification of sinuses, and multiple fractures are encountered. Since the base of the anterior cranial fossa is involved, associated injuries of the brain, CSF leaks, and pneumocephalus may be associated complications and are best evaluated by CT.

Naso-orbital Fractures
The findings are fracture through the frontal bone and nasal bones near the nasofrontal suture, frontal process of the maxillae, lacrimal bones, medial wall of both orbits, cribriform plate, and ethmoid labyrinth. There is widening and depression of the bridge of the nose, with splaying that leads to pseudohypertelorism. Deformity of the medial canthi with injury to the lacrimal drainage system are commonly associated with soft-tissue injuries. Because of these soft-tissue injuries and significant fracture deformities, CT is the preferred method of examination.

Blowout Fractures of the Floor and Medial Wall *(Cases 5–8)*
The blowout fracture of the orbit is the result of a sudden increase in the intraorbital pressure from a blow to the eye. The fracture occurs in the weakest structural portion of the orbit, usually the floor. In about 50 percent of cases, the floor fracture is associated with a medial wall fracture.[8]

The radiographic findings demonstrate the following:

1. downward curvature of the orbital floor
2. bone discontinuity
3. fragmentation with variable displacement of fragments into the maxillary sinus
4. prolapse of orbital contents such as fat and the inferior rectus and inferior oblique muscles into the upper portion of the maxillary antrum
5. opacification with or without a fluid level of the maxillary sinus
6. orbital emphysema from a break of the bone in the medial orbital wall, and rarely floor

On clinical examination, there is ecchymosis about the orbit and lid edema. This may be associated initially with exophthalmos followed by enophthalmos and ptosis of the eyeball as the swelling subsides. The enophthalmos and ptosis of the eyeball result from herniation of orbital contents into the upper third of the antrum through the defect in the orbital floor. Diplopia results from entrapment or prolapse of the inferior oblique and inferior rectus muscles or from hemorrhage and swelling involving the muscles and surrounding fat. There is often infraorbital anesthesia caused by a fracture in the infraorbital canal. Continuity of the orbital floor is restored with a synthetic implant (silastic).

Fracture of the medial wall of the orbit may be isolated or associated with a floor fracture in about 50 percent of cases.[9] Entrapment of the medial rectus muscle is rarely observed. Clinically, the diagnosis of muscle entrapment may be suspected when horizontal diplopia is demonstrated. Muscle entrapment is usually the sequence of an extensive comminuted fracture of the medial wall of the orbit. CT is able to delineate the fracture site, its extent and medial rectus muscle entrapment.[10] In this respect, it is superior to polytomography.

The entity of true muscle entrapment following a blowout fracture has been questioned. Cadaver studies with experimentally produced blowout fractures have revealed a deformity of the inferior rectus muscle that assumes a sharply angulated configuration, without actual incarceration of the muscle by the bony defect.[11] It is postulated that the inferior rectus muscle is pulled down by fibrous bands that attach to the muscle sheath and extend through the posteroinferior fat pad to insert into the periosteum of the orbital floor. As the fat prolapses through the fracture defect, tension is applied via these fibrous bands to the muscle, thereby limiting motion with resultant diplopia in upgaze. There is some clinical evidence to indicate that surgical repair of the fracture defect is not necessary in many of these cases, as in time these fibrous bands will stretch to restore normal motion to the muscles.[12] (See Case 19.)

In view of the linear relationship of the inferior rectus muscle to the orbital floor, a sagittal view is necessary to allow a realistic evaluation of the inferior rectus muscle along its axis. Coronal views alone are inadequate for this purpose.[11] Therefore, blowout fractures of the orbital floor should routinely be studied by sagittal reformations. These are obtained by scanning in the axial plane parallel to the orbital floor, using thin sections (1.5 to 2 mm), from the upper maxillary antrum to the orbital roof. This allows evaluation of the medial orbital wall, as well as provides a basis from which sagittal reformatted views in the plane of the inferior rectus muscle can be made.

Optic Canal Fractures[13] *(Case 9)*

About 1 percent of severe head injuries are associated with impairment of vision.[14] In most instances, the impaired vision results from a fracture of the optic canal. Occasionally, these fractures can be seen on conventional roentgenograms, but transverse tomographic sections perpendicular to the long axis of the optic canal are preferred. A detailed evaluation of the optic canal can be obtained by CT[15] (see Chapter 2). As these are axial views, however, only the medial and lateral walls can be assessed. CT has the advantage of demonstrating soft-tissue damage such as intraorbital optic nerve disruption and hemorrhage. The roof of the optic canal, a frequent site of optic canal fractures, is not adequately evaluated by axial CT sections and may therefore require transverse complex-motion tomography to demonstrate a fracture.

FOREIGN BODIES OF THE EYE AND ORBIT *(Cases 10–18)*

Foreign bodies of the eye and orbit are ophthalmologic emergencies that require thorough evaluation in order to determine an appropriate surgical approach and achieve optimal results. In most cases of ocular trauma, a major diagnostic consideration is the determination of the presence and location of a foreign body. A wide range of imaging techniques is available to assist in screening and localizing foreign bodies. Conventional films are the most widely used. Optical examination is often hampered in patients with severe injury to the globe due to an opacified cornea, opaque anterior media, cataract, or opaque posterior media.

Penetrating eye wounds may be complicated by intraocular hemorrhage, traumatic cataract, detached retina, infection, and decreased vision. Enucleation may become necessary. Intraocular foreign bodies introduce additional risks, including chemical damage such as siderosis from iron and steel, chalcosis from copper, infection (especially from vegetable matter), and mechanical damage such as retinal detachment caused by fibrous adhesions of the retina. The majority of foreign bodies occur on the surface of the cornea, conjunctiva, or anterior sclera and are usually removed in the emergency ward. This may be achieved by irrigation or may require instrument extraction with needles or forceps, usually performed under local anesthesia. Intraocular foreign bodies are removed by various ophthalmologic procedures. Orbital foreign bodies are usually not removed unless they interfere with the motion of the globe or cause infection. Most orbital foreign bodies—including metal such as iron, steel, and copper—are inert.

Conventional films are effective in imaging most intraocular foreign bodies. Such success is attributable to the fact that most objects that occur clinically as intraocular foreign bodies are metal.[16] In addition, most objects with sufficient momentum to penetrate the globe are greater than 1 mm in their largest dimension. Conventional films readily give images of pieces of iron, steel, or other metal 0.5 mm or greater in diameter. However, pieces of stone, aluminum, and glass without significant lead content that are smaller than 1.5 mm and organic materials such as wood are not visualized on conventional films. In these instances, CT by virtue of its sensitivity is able to visualize low-density or radiolucent foreign bodies.[1,2,17] Manipulation of the window width may assist in the detection of a foreign body; the ideal window width setting is 500 H units, with a level of 50 H units. Computerized tomography can demonstrate copper and steel with a minimal detectable size of 0.06 mm[3].[18] The minimum volumes for detectable aluminum in this reported series were 25 times greater. Wood fragments were not reliably detected.

From the management point of view, it is important to determine the relationship of the foreign body to the globe and to establish whether it is intra- or extraocular. This can often be demonstrated by utilizing axial and coronal CT sections. The relationship of the foreign body to the optic nerve is similarly of clinical importance and can be determined by axial and coronal studes.

Introduction of a foreign body associated with trauma may be unnoticed by the patient, and there may be considerable delay of weeks or months before diagnosis. Sharp foreign bodies may penetrate the soft-tissue structures of the orbit and cause relatively small entrance wounds. It is often to the surprise of the ophthalmologist to find a large foreign body embedded in the deep portion of the orbit. Sharp objects may penetrate the roof of the orbit and enter the intracranial cavity, where complications such as a brain abscess may develop.

The use of CT in the diagnosis of foreign bodies is limited in the following situations. Low-density objects such as wood and other vegetable matter may not be visualized. A foreign body may be concealed by a surrounding hemorrhage, inflammatory exudate, abscess, or granuloma. A dense, metallic foreign body, especially if large, causes disturbing artifacts that may degrade the image sufficiently to preclude precise local-

ization of the foreign body relative to the globe or optic nerve.

EXPERIMENTAL BLOWOUT FRACTURES
(Case 19)

Experimental blowout fractures are illustrated in Case 19.

REFERENCES

1. Grove A: Orbital trauma evaluation by computed tomography. Comput Tomog 3:267–278, 1979
2. Grove A: Orbital trauma and computed tomography. Ophthalmology (Rochester) 87:403–411, 1980
3. Rowe LD, Miller E, Brant-Zawadzki M: Computed tomography in maxillofacial trauma. Laryngoscope 91:745–751, 1981
4. Espagno J, Manelfe C, Bousigue JY, et al: The usefulness and prognostic value of CT scanning in cranio-cerebral trauma. J Neuroradiol 7:121–132, 1980
5. Saul TG, Ducker TB: The role of computed tomography in acute head injury. CT 4:296–308, 1980
6. Ghoshhajra K: CT in trauma of the base of the skull and its complications. CT 4:271–276, 1980.
7. Merrick R, Latchaw R, Gold L: Computerized tomography of the orbit in carotid-cavernous sinus fistulae. Comput Tomog 4:127–132, 1980
8. Converse JM, Smith B: Orbital blow-out fractures: a ten-year survey. Plast Reconstr Surg 39:20–36, 1967
9. Hammerschlag SB, Hughes S, O'Reilly GV, Weber AL: Another look at blowout fractures. AJNR 3:331–335, 1982
10. Zilkha A: Computed tomography of blow-out fractures of the medial orbital wall. AJNR 2:427–429, 1981
11. Hammerschlag SB, Hughes S, O'Reilly GV, et al: Blowout fractures of the orbit: a comparison of computed tomography and conventional radiography with anatomical correlation. Radiology 143:487–492, 1982
12. Putterman AM, Stevens T, Urist MJ: Nonsurgical management of blowout fractures of the orbital floor. Am J Ophthal 77:232–239, 1974
13. Ramsay JH: Optic nerve injury in fracture of the canal. Br J Ophthalmol 63:607–610, 1979
14. Lombardi G: Radiology in Neuro-ophthalmology. Baltimore, Williams & Wilkins, p 506, 1967
15. Hammerschlag SB, O'Reilly GV, Naheedy MH: Computed tomography of the optic canals. AJNR 2:593–594, 1981
16. Duke-Elder WS: Systems of Ophthalmology, Vol 14, Part I, St. Louis, CV Mosby, pp 477–544, 1958
17. Gaster RN, Duda EE: Localization of intraocular foreign bodies by computed tomography. Ophthalmic Surg 11(1):25–29, 1980
18. Tate E, Cupples H: Detection of orbital foreign bodies with computed tomography. Am J Neuroradiol 2:363–365, 1981

CASE 1. Tripod Fracture of the Zygoma with an Orbital Floor Fracture
This patient sustained a blow to the right side of the face.

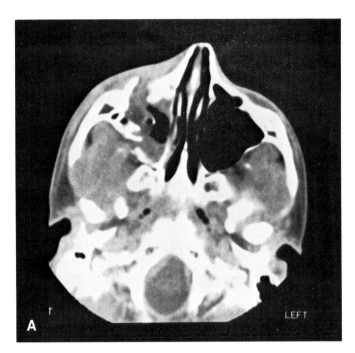

Figure A. A scan through the maxillary sinuses demonstrates fractures of the anterior and lateral walls of the right maxillary sinus. Other sections demonstrated a fracture of the zygomatic arch as well. There is considerable soft-tissue swelling within the antrum. Also noted is increased soft-tissue density in the infratemporal fossa, representing associated hematoma.

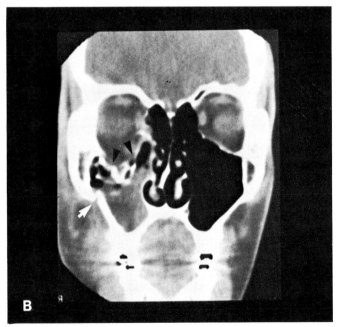

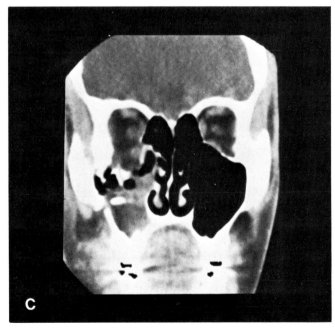

Figures B and C. Coronal scans demonstrate a large fracture (arrowheads) of the floor of the right orbit. Bony fragments are displaced inferiorly into the right antrum, and there is near-complete opacification of the antrum. Again noted is the fracture of the lateral wall of the antrum (arrow).

CASE 2. Orbital Fractures

This 46-year-old male had a history of a left skull fracture with CSF rhinor-rhea that required a craniotomy for repair. He was also blind in the left eye as a result of that accident. Recently, the patient was struck in the left eye with a wood post, which resulted in left enophthalmos and complete ptosis of the left upper lid.

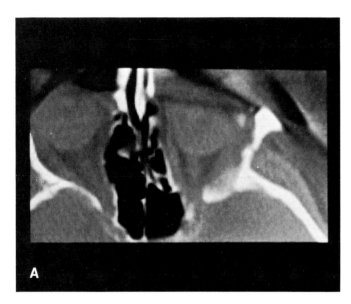 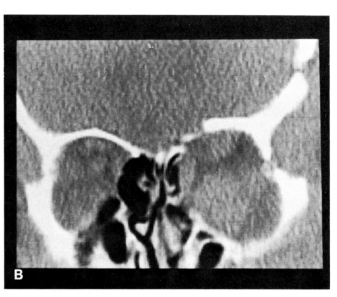

Figures A and B. Axial and coronal scans demonstrate fractures of the roof, lateral wall, and floor of the left orbit. On the coronal scan, the zygoma is noted to be displaced laterally and inferiorly. There is also a fracture of the left frontal bone. There is a blowout fracture of the medial wall of the orbit with displacement of the lamina papyracea into the left ethmoid sinuses. Presumably, the recent injury caused the blowout fracture, which in turn resulted in enophthalmos.

CASE 3. LeFort III Fracture

The patient was involved in a motorcycle accident. On clinical examination there was marked swelling of the face and bilateral proptosis. The exam was also suggestive of cranial facial separation.

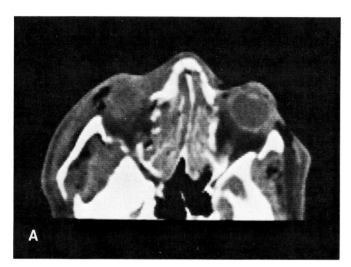 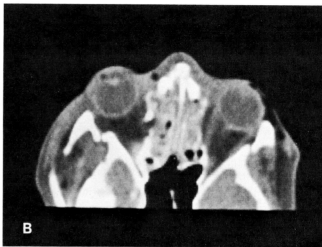

Figures A and B. There is complete opacification of the ethmoid sinuses with multiple fractures of the ethmoid. Also noted are fractures of the lateral walls of both orbits. Air is present within the subcutaneous tissues surrounding the orbits. The globes are proptotic. No retrobulbar hematoma is evident.

Follow-up: There was no serious ocular injury. Plain films and polytomes confirmed a LeFort III fracture.

CASE 4. Complex LeFort III Fracture
This 19-year-old male was in an automobile accident and received multiple facial injuries.

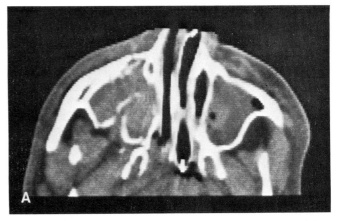

Figure A. A scan through the maxillary sinuses shows fractures of anterior and posterior walls of the right antrum. Bone fragments are seen within the sinus and the sinus is completely opacified. Also noted is considerable swelling of the soft tissues in the nasopharynx.

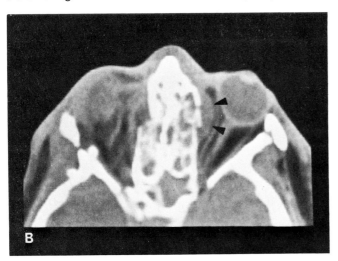

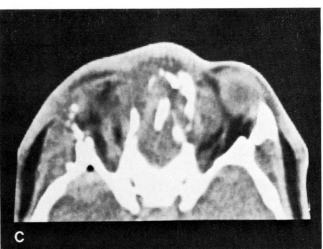

Figures B and C. Sections through the orbits demonstrate comminuted fractures of the ethmoid sinuses and perpendicular plate. Also noted are fractures of the lateral walls of both orbits. There is gross distortion of architecture of the right orbit, with anterior and inferior displacement of the globe and considerable hemorrhage anteriorly and in the extraconal spaces. The left globe is also proptotic. A subperiosteal hematoma (arrowheads) displaces the medial rectus muscle laterally. The ethmoid and sphenoid sinuses are completely opacified.

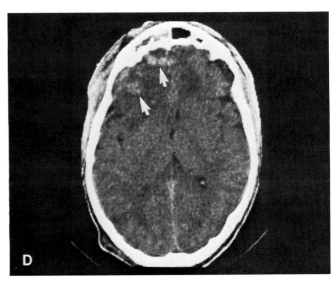

Figure D. There are hemorrhagic contusions (arrows) involving both frontal lobes, more marked on the right side. Also noted is opacification of the right frontal sinus.

CASE 5. Blowout Fractures of the Right Orbit

This patient suffered a blow to the right orbit. Plain films revealed no evidence of fracture. Vision and extraocular movements were normal.

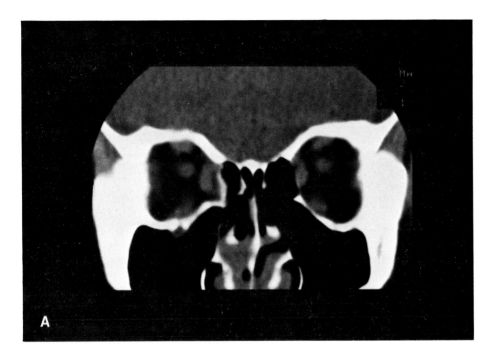

Figure A. A coronal scan reveals medial displacement of the lamina papyracea, as well as a focal depression of the floor of the right orbit. No other abnormalities are noted.

CASE 6. Medial Blowout Fracture

This is a 61-year-old female who was in a motor vehicle accident and sustained multiple facial injuries. On physical examination the patient had diplopia and left enophthalmos.

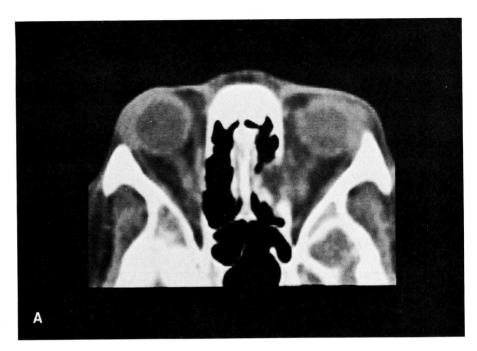

Figure A. There is a blowout fracture of the medial wall of the left orbit. Soft-tissue density protrudes into the adjacent ethmoid sinuses. Soft-tissue density is also present in the medial orbit, probably representing some hemorrhage. The course of the medial rectus muscle cannot be followed through the soft-tissue density.

CASE 7. Blowout Fracture

This 58-year-old male injured his right eye during a fall. He noted occasional double vision when looking up. On clinical examination there was right enophthalmos and ptosis of the globe with limited upward gaze.

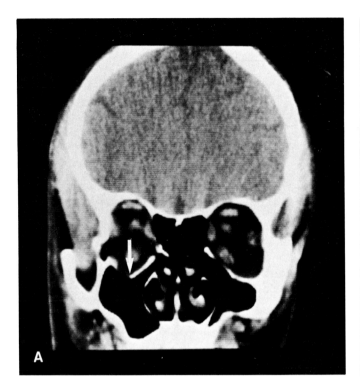 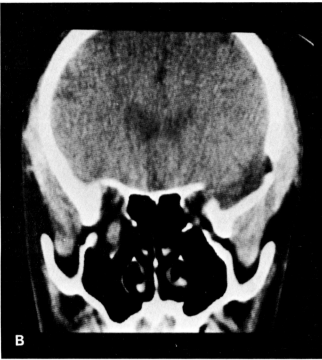

Figures A and B. Coronal scans demonstrate a blowout fracture of the floor of the right orbit with inferior depression of the bony fragments (arrow) and contents of the right orbit. Also noted is medial displacement of the lamina papyracea, indicating a medial blowout fracture as well.

Follow-up: At surgery the prolapsed orbital soft tissues were reduced and the bony defect was covered with a prosthesis. Following surgery the eye assumed an almost normal horizontal position, and the patient noted considerable improvement in the double vision.

CASE 8. Blowout Fractures Treated with an Orbital Plate

A blow to this patient's right eye resulted in blowout fractures of the right orbit. A plate was inserted into the floor of the orbit to give support to the orbital structures.

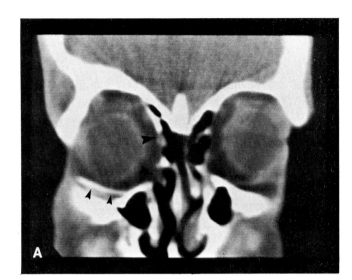 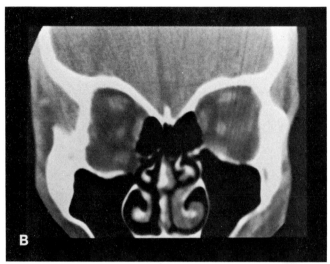

Figures A and B. There is a blowout fracture of the floor of the right orbit with inferior depression of the bony wall. A plate (small arrowheads) is evident below the right globe. Also noted is a blowout fracture of the medial wall (large arrowheads) with displacement of the bony margins into the adjacent ethmoid sinuses. The right globe remains in a slightly inferior position relative to the left. The residual enophthalmos is apparently due to an unrepaired medial defect together with residual prolapse through the posterior aspect of the floor defect in B. The prosthetic plate has not been placed sufficiently posteriorly in the orbit to cover the entire floor fracture.

CASE 9. Fracture of the Optic Canal
This patient had trauma to the left side of the face.

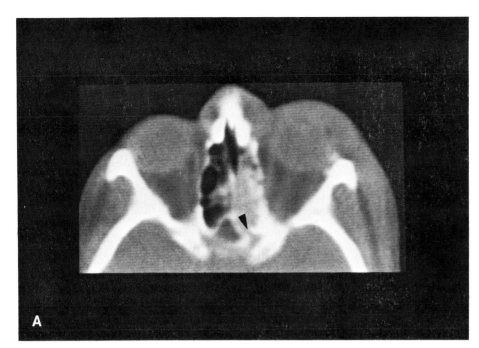

A

Figure A. There are multiple fractures of the left ethmoid with the fractures extending into the lamina papyracea in multiple areas. The left ethmoid sinuses are opacified. Also noted is a fracture of the medial wall of the left optic canal (arrowhead). There is also considerable soft-tissue swelling about the anterior aspect of the left orbit.

CASE 10. Gunshot Wound to the Right Orbit

This 34-year-old female received a gunshot wound to the right orbit. She presented with increasing proptosis and chemosis of the lids. She had no residual vision in the right eye; vision in the left eye was normal.

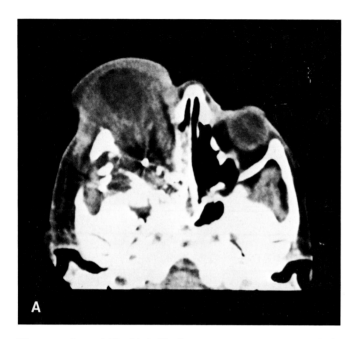 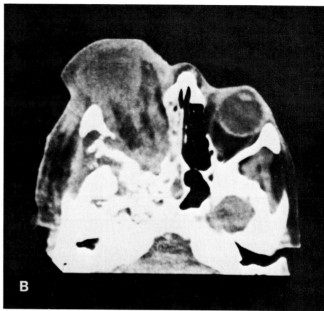

Figures A and B. Metallic fragments are present within the right orbit, temporal fossa, and base of skull. Multiple additional fragments were present in the maxillary sinus and middle fossa. There are fractures of the lateral wall of the orbit and the base of skull. The lamina papyracea is fractured and displaced medially into the ethmoid sinuses. The globe is markedly proptotic and soft-tissue density surrounding the globe represents hematoma. The medial and lateral rectus muscles are also edematous.

Follow-up: Polytomes revealed an additional stellate fracture of the right petrous bone. An arteriogram revealed a pseudoaneurysm of the right internal carotid artery associated with a carotid cavernous fistula. This was treated with intraarterial balloon occlusion of the fistula and the right carotid artery. Due to the severe injury to the right orbit, enucleation and partial exenteration of the right eye and anterior orbit were necessary.

CASE 11. Penetrating Injury of the Globe

This 26-year-old male was raking material from the floor at work when he heard an explosive noise, followed by pain in the right eye. On physical examination, he had lacerations of both the upper and lower lids and a penetrating injury through the cornea and iris.

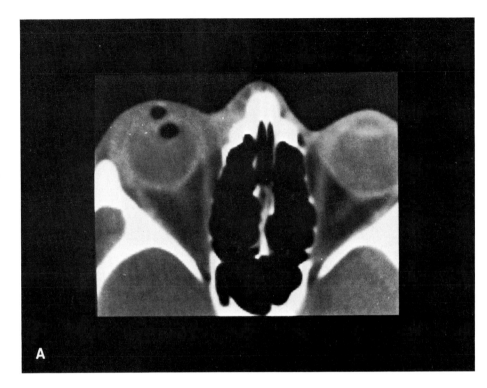

A

Figure A. An axial scan shows air within the anterior and posterior chambers of the right eye. No foreign body is identified. There is associated soft-tissue swelling of the anterior orbital structures.

Follow-up: The patient underwent a corneal-scleral repair with excision of iris fragments. The upper and lower lid lacerations were also repaired. The hyphema of the right eye slowly cleared, but the vision in the right eye consisted of light perception. Postoperatively, he had severe pain OD and after one week he had no vision in the right eye. Because of the persistent pain, an enucleation was performed.

CASE 12. Foreign Body in Apex of Orbit
This 14-year-old male was injured from a shotgun blast. The pellets hit the ground and deflected into his face.

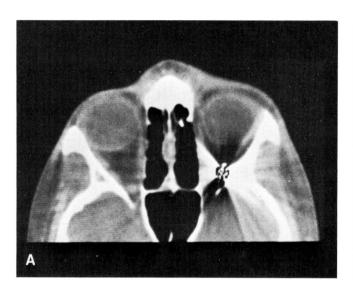
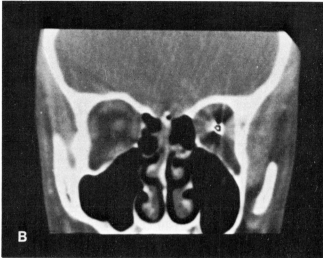

Figures A and B. Axial and coronal scans show a metallic foreign body in the apex of the left orbit. Artifacts from the foreign body obscure anatomical detail. The foreign body is positioned lateral to the optic nerve.

Follow-up: The patient initially had some diplopia, edema, and ecchymosis of his eyelids, all of which resolved during the first week. On follow-up examination six months later, a permanent choroidal scar was noted in the left eye. Vision was 20/20 OD and 20/25 OS, and the patient had normal eye movements. Due to the posterior location of the foreign body and the patient's normal vision, the foreign body was not removed.

CASE 13. Intraocular Foreign Body OD

This 11-year-old male was struck in the right eye while hitting a metal wedge with a sledge hammer. Examination revealed a corneal laceration and cataract.

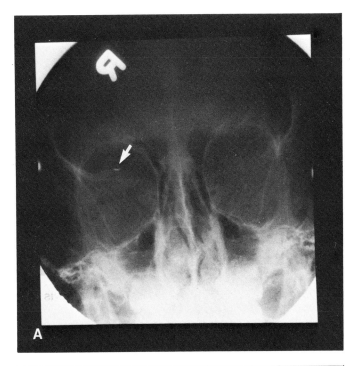

Figure A. A plain film of the orbits shows a small, metallic foreign body projected over the right orbit (arrow). The sinuses are normally aerated.

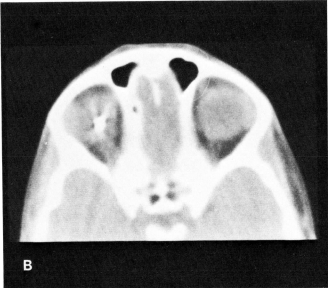

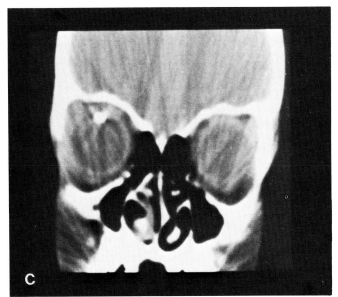

Figures B and C. Axial and coronal scans demonstrate a metallic foreign body in the sclera of the right eye at about 12 o'clock.

Follow-up: The patient underwent emergency surgery for repair of the corneal laceration and a lensectomy OD. A second operation was performed to remove the intraocular foreign body and for a scleral buckle procedure.

CASE 14. Foreign Body in the Left Eye
This 40-year-old male was seen a week after he received a penetrating injury to the left eye. Physical examination showed conjunctival and episcleral injection but no foreign body.

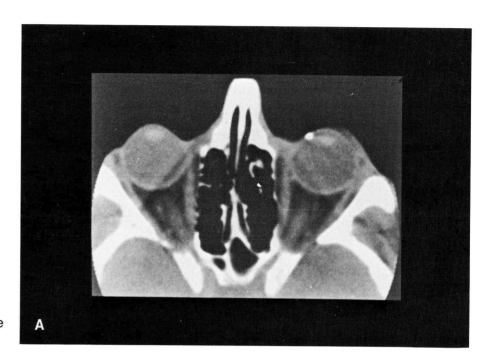

Figure A. CT scan shows a foreign body that is either on or within the sclera just medial to the corneal-scleral junction (limbus).

A

Follow-up: Orbital ultrasound determined the foreign body to be either within the sclera or the adjacent ciliary body. At surgery, a 1-mm entrance wound was found parallel to the limbus at a 10 o'clock position. The metallic foreign body was embedded in the ciliary body.

CASE 15. Foreign Body in the Right Orbit

This 48-year-old male felt something strike his eye while operating a jackhammer. When he arrived at the emergency room, the left globe was severely proptotic and displaced inferiorly. A retrobulbar hemorrhage was diagnosed and promptly drained with a needle. Following aspiration, the proptosis was reduced and the extraocular movements were much improved. A CT scan was then done to localize the foreign body.

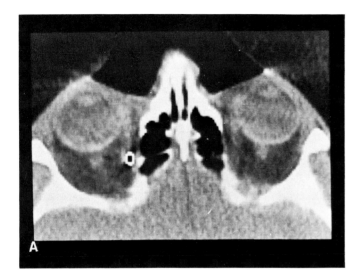 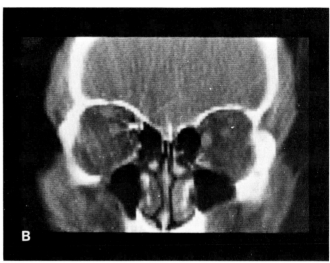

Figures A and B. Axial and coronal scans reveal a metallic foreign body in the medial extraconal space of the right orbit adjacent to the medial rectus muscle. The globe is in normal position and no residual orbital hematoma is evident.

Follow-up: The patient was treated with antibiotics, but the foreign body was not removed.

CASE 16. BB Shot in the Right Orbit
This 22-year-old male was shot in the right orbit with a BB gun at 25 yards. Clinical examination revealed a rupture of the globe, but the foreign body was not identified.

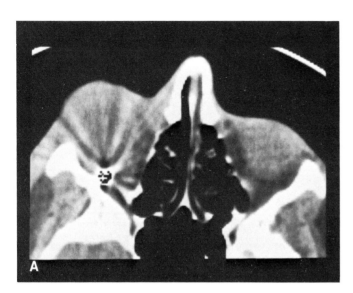 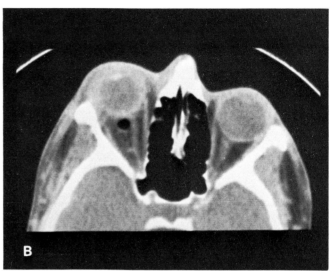

Figure A. There is a metallic foreign body in the lateral retrobulbar space of the right orbit. It lies beneath the lateral rectus muscle. The ethmoid and sphenoid sinuses are clear.

Figure B. On a higher section, the right globe is proptotic. A locule of air lies behind the globe lateral to the optic nerve. The rim of the globe is thickened, and there is a slight increase in the overall density of the vitreous chamber.

Follow-up: Ultrasound confirmed the foreign body in the lateral right orbit. Also noted was massive vitreous hemorrhage and possible retinal detachment. The patient was then taken to surgery for repair of the ruptured globe and excision of prolapsed uvea. A follow-up surgical procedure was required one week later, at which time a pars plana vitrectomy, lensectomy, and scleral buckle procedure were done.

CASE 17. Foreign Body in the Left Orbit

While hunting, this 31-year-old male was struck in the left cheek and left medial canthus with two shotgun pellets. Upon admission to the emergency room, retinal and choroidal rupture was noted. He then underwent a cryopexy of the retinal hole and a scleral buckling procedure. A CT scan was performed at a later date to localize the foreign body.

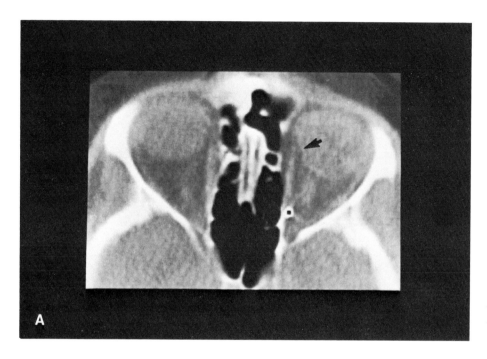

Figure A. There is a metallic foreign body measuring approximately 2 mm in diameter in the posterior medial aspect of the left orbit. The foreign body is either within the medial rectus muscle or in the intraconal space. The deformity of the posterior medial globe (arrow) probably represents the site of penetration of the globe and the region of the scleral buckling procedure.

CASE 18. Intraocular Foreign Body

This eight-year-old female was struck in the left eye with metal fragments when her brother fired a rifle at a rock. She was seen at a local hospital and the diagnosis of corneal abrasion was made. She was given an eye ointment to use four times a day. Two days later, she came to the emergency room with increasing redness and blurry vision in the left eye. Upon admission, her visual acuity was 20/25 OD and OS was counting fingers in the temporal periphery. A small corneal foreign body was seen at 8 o'clock midway to the limbus.

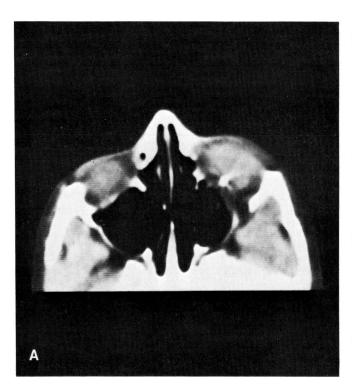 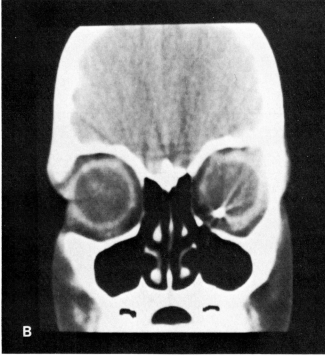

Figures A and B. Axial and coronal scans reveal a metallic foreign body in the inferior medial aspect of the globe immediately adjacent to the sclera. The adjacent sinuses are normally aerated.

Follow-up: Following an anterior chamber tap, the patient underwent a lensectomy, vitrectomy, and removal of the foreign body. A scleral buckle procedure was also performed.

CASE 19. Experimental Blowout Fractures*

Blowout fractures were created in cadaver orbits with subsequent CT scanning in the direct oblique sagittal plane (parallel to the long axis of the inferior rectus muscle).

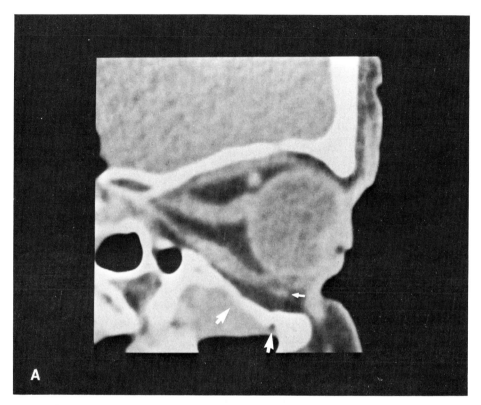

Figure A. A blowout fracture of the orbital floor is present (large arrows) with no significant depression. The configuration of the inferior rectus muscle and the inferior oblique muscle (small arrow) is normal. The posteroinferior orbital fat pad below the muscles is normal. Fluid is present in the maxillary antrum (vertex down position). Mobility of the inferior rectus muscle on forced duction testing was normal.

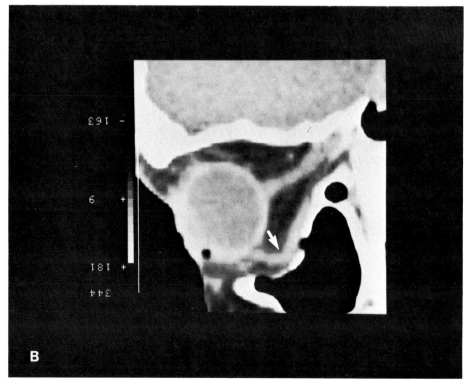

Figure B. Blowout fracture of the orbital floor with a depressed segment. There is mild angulation of the depressed inferior rectus muscle (arrow). The forced duction test was normal.

*Reprinted from Hammerschlag SB, Hughes S, O'Reilly GV, et al: Blow-out fractures of the orbit: a comparison of computed tomography and conventional radiography with anatomical correlation. Radiology 143:487–492, 1982, with permission.

continued

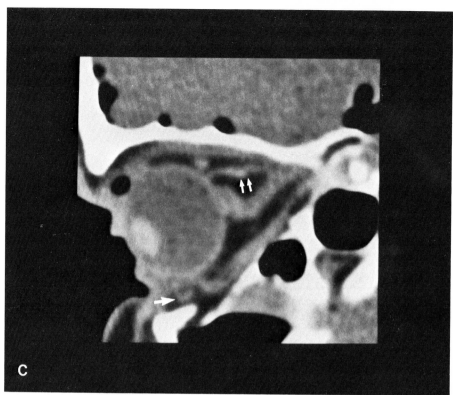

Figure C. Blowout fracture of the orbital floor. Orbital fat from the inferior orbital fat pad has prolapsed through the defect, and there is angulation of the inferior rectus muscle above the prolapsed fat. The forced duction test was equivocal. The inferior oblique muscle (arrow) is intact. Note the marked enophthalmos, due primarily to a large medial wall blowout fracture with prolapse into the ethmoid labyrinth. Incidentally, note the superior ophthalmic vein (double arrows).

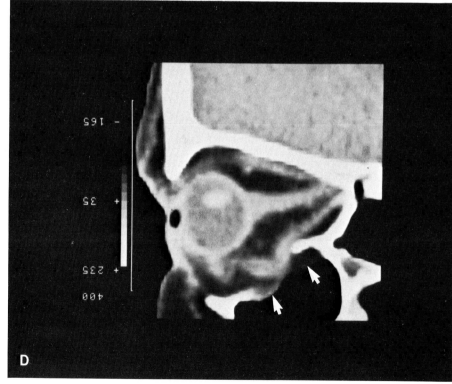

Figure D. Blowout fracture of the orbital floor, with a sharply kinked inferior rectus muscle prolapsing through the defect in the floor. The bony margin of the defect, however, does not abut the inferior rectus muscle anteriorly, indicating that the muscle itself is not incarcerated by bone. The forced duction test was positive, and this is thought to be secondary to significant prolapse of the inferior orbital fat pad (arrows) below and adjacent to the inferior rectus muscle. Note the dislocation of the ocular lens secondary to the trauma.

Index